Penguin Health
Immunity Plus

Arabella Melville was born in Cheshire in 1948. She graduated
in psychology at the University of Birmingham and was awarded
a Ph.D. in 1974. After a period as a research assistant at McGill
University, Montreal, she worked as a feature writer, producing
articles on popular psychology and health topics for magazines
and newspapers, including *Cosmopolitan* and the *Liverpool Daily
Post*. From 1978 until 1981 she was research assistant at the
Medical Sociology Research Centre, University College, Swan-
sea, and published several papers on her findings. During this
period she began writing her first book and, since 1981, has
been a full-time author, writing books and articles on health and
related topics mainly in collaboration with her partner, Colin
Johnson. She has published numerous articles in newspapers,
including the *Observer* and the *Guardian*, and in magazines,
including *New Health*, *New Society*, *Cosmopolitan*, *Woman* and
General Practitioner, and she is a regular reviewer of papers on
prescribing submitted to *Social Science and Medicine*. She also
broadcasts and lectures widely, mainly on the subjects of drug
use and health.

Colin Johnson was born in 1939 in Essex. His first job was as a
garage mechanic. He went on to tool-making and then to drafting
and design. He studied for a HNC in Mechanical Engineering
and became a consultant designer. He made major contributions
to the development of the industrial co-operative movement in
the early 1960s and eventually started up his own business in
distribution. After a brief return to consultancy in the 1970s he
began writing on questions of health with Arabella Melville.
The books they have jointly written include *Cured to Death: The
Effects of Prescription Drugs* (1982), *Hay Fever: No Need to Suffer*
(1984), *The Long-life Heart: How to Avoid Heart Disease and Live a
Longer Life* (1985), *Persistent Fat and How to Lose It* (1986) and
Alternatives to Drugs (1987). Colin Johnson is director of Life
Profile Ltd, a personal health advisory service, and Health Information Services, a company that provides detailed briefings on
specific topics for corporate and media clients. He also lectures
widely on health and ecology.

Arabella Melville and
Colin Johnson

IMMUNITY PLUS

*How to be Healthy in the
Age of New Infections*

PENGUIN BOOKS

PENGUIN BOOKS

Published by the Penguin Group
27 Wrights Lane, London W8 5TZ, England
Viking Penguin Inc., 40 West 23rd Street, New York, New York 10010, USA
Penguin Books Australia Ltd, Ringwood, Victoria, Australia
Penguin Books Canada Ltd, 2801 John Street, Markham, Ontario, Canada L3R 1B4
Penguin Books (NZ) Ltd, 182–190 Wairau Road, Auckland 10, New Zealand

Penguin Books Ltd, Registered Offices: Harmondsworth, Middlesex, England

First published 1988

Copyright © Arabella Melville and Colin Johnson, 1988
Illustrations by Andrew Farmer
All rights reserved

Made and printed in Great Britain by
Richard Clay Ltd, Bungay, Suffolk
Filmset in Monophoto 10/12 Palatino

Contents

Preface

Of all the events which mark human history, the emergence of infectious scourges leaves the deepest impression. The passing of kings, even of great wars, fades with time, but the Black Death and the Great Plague still strike a chill chord in our collective memory. Today we face the challenge of another infectious scourge which could similarly scar the consciousness of our species.

AIDS has the potential for changing the course of human development. While nothing which causes misery and death is welcome, the lesson of history is that we can respond positively to tragedy. The nature of the changes precipitated by AIDS will depend upon whether we can defeat the cause or be forced to learn to live with it. For the foreseeable future we all have to live with it; even if a vaccine is found, it will take some time, perhaps decades, to eradicate the virus.

In the age of AIDS, we all need to change the way we think about health. While infectious diseases are having a resurgence, to remain healthy we have to act to resist *all* infectious diseases. Once we become the victim of one infection, we are more likely to succumb to others.

Improving immunity is relatively easy. This book will explain, in straightforward and practical terms, how the complicated human immune system works, what we can do to enhance its operation, and what disrupts its efficiency. When medicine has no answer, positive action of this sort is the only sensible course.

Ultimately, as new disease entities emerge, survival may depend upon changing the way we think. This change has occurred with other types of disease. Heart-disease fatalities have dropped as people change their lifestyles, for it has been accepted that much of the disease can be avoided by thinking in the right way and making appropriate choices.

With hidden threats, such as AIDS, we need to adopt both the right attitude and the right action. In addition, since we will not always be able to avoid infections, we also need to ensure that we live in ways which will enhance our immunity. With AIDS the attitude we must adopt is that *everyone* could have the virus, and we need to behave accordingly. Gays and drug addicts may have fallen victim to AIDS first, not directly because of their exposure to the virus (although exposure among these groups was high), but because promiscuity and drug abuse damage and compromise the immune system. These cultural sub-groups are much more liable to suffer from other infections for exactly the same reason.

The lesson is clear. We must all do whatever is needed to improve our resistance to infections. This will make us healthier, and healthy people limit the spread of all illness. There is no other choice.

Because we are all different and our degree of susceptibility to illness varies widely, there is no single simple-minded answer to the problem of creating health. Improving your immunity, and creating lasting health, depends first upon getting the basics right. Once these are established, you can use your experience and knowledge to modify the subtle factors which are relevant to you as a unique individual. The recommendations we make will spell out the basics and give you insight into possible further requirements.

Diseases are changing and evolving all the time. If we stand still, we will be overcome and will fail. The winning strategy, for all of us, is not to wait passively for 'others' to find that single simple-minded answer, for most such answers are illusory. We progress against disease by consolidating the hard-won lessons of the past, of hygiene, nutrition, lifestyle and behaviour; we have to add further sound structure to these foundations. Waiting for medicine is a last resort; our elevation of it to first and only resort may be seen historically as a trap. Those waiting for medicine today may find it arrives too late. With improved immunity, and generally increased health, you will find that medicine becomes your last resort. When you use it rarely, its minimal intervention brings more benefit.

Your immune system protects you all the time. Its ceaseless and automatic action is easy to overlook, to take for granted. We hope when you have read *Immunity Plus* you will be filled with wonder and determination – wonder at the competence and complexity of the battle, for that is what it is, within you, and determination to do all you can to help the goodies win.

PART 1

THE BATTLE FOR YOUR BODY

Plato described health as 'a love affair between the organs of the body'. Like all such relationships, health is at constant risk of disruption — from enemies without, from conditions imposed upon it, and from mistakes made within.

In the battle for your body, medicine and its various specialists tend to concentrate on the front-line troops. They are important, for we would have no immunity without battalions of white cells, complements, antibodies, Natural Killers, and so on. But wars are won by industry. No matter how grand their uniforms, how splendid their drill, or how clever their plans, if soldiers are not supplied with weapons, fuel and ammunition, they cannot fight. They may gallantly win the odd battle, but eventually they will be overwhelmed.

Our approach to improving immunity assumes that the troops know their jobs and can be left to get on with them as required. We will concentrate on directing the way you live, so that they are well supplied, are available in sufficient numbers and, crucially, the capacity of their back-up is adequate to meet the demands that pathogens put upon the system. We start with the body's industrial capacity, the efficiency of its metabolism.

Immunity is a complex subject; many of its fine details are still being explored. Our objective is not so much to explain this complexity, as to give a series of pictures which will enable you to understand what is important in improving the overall function of your immune system. To be successful you need to know how to organize your body so that its response is appropriate, and your health retained.

We use a series of diagrams to explain the battle for your body. As with all battle plans, they only show a part of the picture. In all wars many things happen at once; there is much chaos and apparent confusion. Diagrams are static; they cannot show the dynamics of what is actually happening in reality. We hope your imagination will fill in the gaps and bring the picture alive for you.

Once you have such a picture you can exert influence over the battle. You can do the right thing without having to know what happens right down to the front line. Just as when driving you change gear to alter your speed without understanding how a syncromesh works (or even what it is), so you can affect health or illness by understanding what to do, without needing to understand details of microbiology.

Some areas of disease and immunity will need examination in detail. There will be times when influence at the molecular level will be crucial to the outcome of the situation as a whole, when small details have a disproportionate effect on the outcome. When necessary, we will pursue these details, without losing sight of the larger picture.

This integrated approach is essential. Our culture encourages us to believe that every problem has a single simple answer. The truth is that illness is a complex problem, and the battle we fight against it equally complex. The action we take to influence the battle has to complement this complexity. With your picture of what is involved in improving immunity, and knowledge of your own situation, you will be able to do this. These positive strategies will do much to ensure that the battle for your body will not turn into war, and that most of the time peace will prevail.

Boosting Immunity:
A Strategy for Health

Our immune systems are complex and beautiful examples of biological adaptability. They evolved with us over millions of years, as we clashed with many other creatures pursuing their own evolutionary paths. Immunity protects us against invasion and takeover by a wide range of potential enemies.

In our shared global environment, every life-form depends upon others for its survival. Higher life-forms crop or kill and eat those lower down the scale. Many lower forms fight back, killing much more complex plants and animals, as all seek to extend their command of global resources. Humans are not excluded from these life-cycles: we are under attack from hundreds of microscopic life-forms all the time.

The degree to which one life-form is able to resist the attacks of others creates the balance of life. The total interaction is figuratively described as the web of life; its balance will alter from time to time, as environments change, species evolve, decline or outgrow their resources. Even during the most stable epochs, inter-species conflicts finely hone each other, removing the weaker individuals for the benefit of all. Although we may not like it, the failure of the weak and the survival of the strong is one of nature's primary mechanisms. Another is its way of dealing with the over-strong: those species which overextend themselves tend to fall through the web and fail.

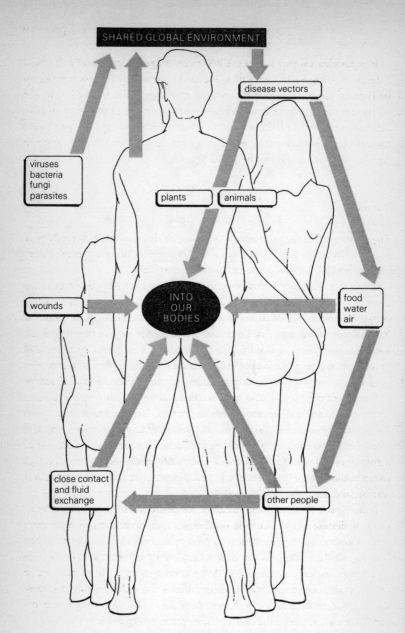

Figure 1

It is paradoxical that humans, some of the largest and certainly the most extended of the Earth's creatures, suffer so much from the unwanted attentions of some of the planet's smallest creatures. Indeed, they live in and on us in colonies all the time. Trouble arises when we cannot maintain our defences, or when we lack the capacity to deal with new types or pathogens from different environments, as when a new 'flu virus evolves or we go to another region of the world for a holiday.

Vectors

To see how pathogens affect us, let us imagine that you are a perfectly pure person, uncontaminated by any other life-forms. How do you become colonized by hosts of viruses, bacteria, fungi and parasites?

The general answer is that they come into contact with us because we share the same environment; indeed, many of them are an integral part of our environment. Even before we are born, we pick up both pathogens and immunity from our mothers. Once out of the womb, we live together in the same biological envelope of the planet. Pathogens have a variety of ways of getting on and into our bodies. These routes, which may involve a variety of other life-forms, or the contamination of food and drink, are called *vectors*.

From the amorphous global environment it is sometimes possible to focus right down to a single very specific disease vector. The best-known example is the possibility of worm infestation from undercooked pork; properly cooked meat creates no problem. Our first line of defence against any disease is to disrupt its vectors and prevent the causative organism from getting through to our bodies. To do this we need a broad understanding of the routes used by disease, and the factors which are important in their management.

From Figure 2 you will see that there are possibilities for complex interactions of disease vectors outside our bodies. Pathogens may occupy more than one clear-cut vector, they may spill over from one to others as they become more common, they may adapt and transfer from one to another, as if seeking the best route in. It would be an exaggeration to ascribe such a tactical purpose to them, but in the end this is the picture which develops. Microscopic pathogens are both persistent and prolific; by weight of numbers they are able to fill the opportunities presented to them.

The other thing you will notice from Figure 2 is that the outcome of

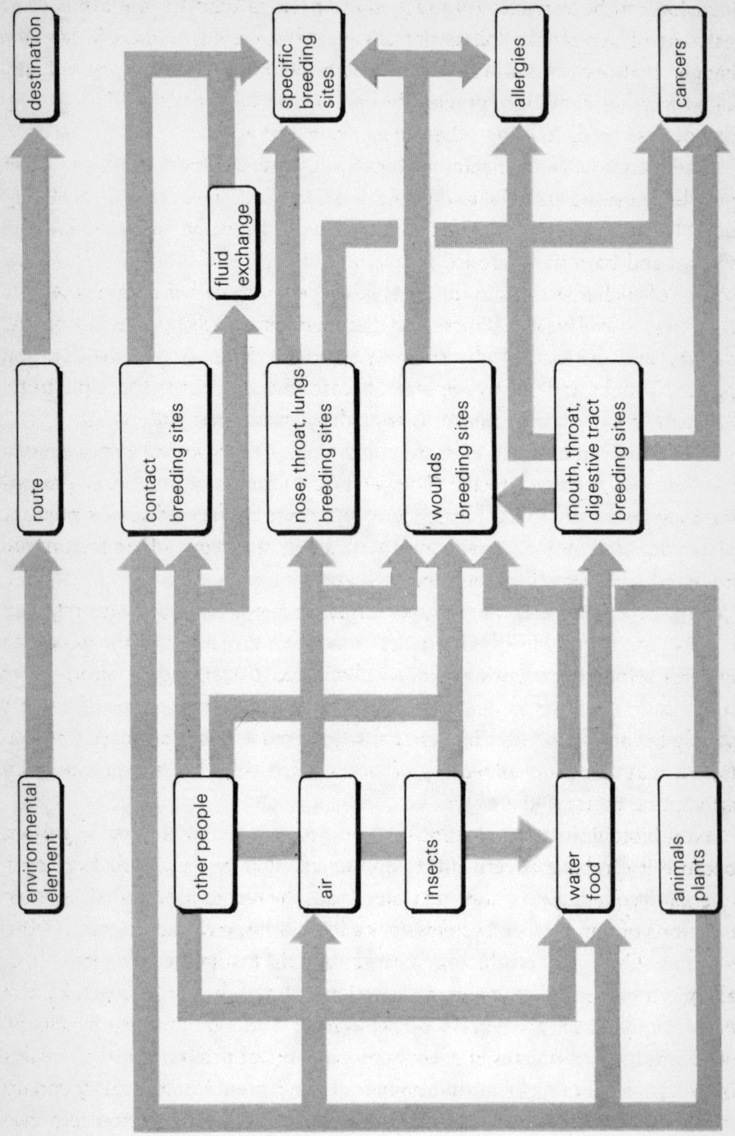
destination
specific breeding sites
allergies
cancers
fluid exchange
route
contact breeding sites
nose, throat, lungs breeding sites
wounds breeding sites
mouth, throat, digestive tract breeding sites
environmental element
other people
air
insects
water food
animals plants

Figure 2

invasion can be variable. Although some bacteria tend to produce specific patterns of symptoms, this is not always what we experience. It can also happen that one virus attack may be fought off, but the damage caused may allow another condition, previously held in check, to emerge. This is why one disease tends to bring others along in its wake.

There are four fundamental vectors for disease: air, food, drink and other people. These are essential to the continuation of our lives and are constantly open to pathogens. Most infections are caught from the air; we breathe in viruses and bacteria cocooned in microscopic drops of moisture. The usual source of such infections in the air is other people; weather maps show how they may travel vast distances, but their virulence will be affected by the density and distance of the source population. The old health-education poster 'Coughs and Sneezes Spread Diseases' has the virtue of simple truth, but merely sharing the same air is enough to share some pathogens.

Our food can also act as host to infections. When we eat contaminated food we *may* become infected. The periodic outbreaks of salmonella poisoning bear testimony to the efficiency of this route from the disease's point of view. But it is not a certain means of infection; many other factors are involved apart from ingesting the pathogen.

Similarly, water and other drinks can carry infectious organisms into our bodies. The World Health Organization believes that much of the disease in underdeveloped countries could be eliminated by providing clean water supplies. In countries in decline or suffering population overload, the water supply becomes suspect. This is not always because of biological contamination; it may also happen because of increasing chemical pollution caused by attempting to 'treat' the water.

Non-biological contamination of these basic vectors is very important because it can have severe effects on our immune systems. Pollution, both overt and covert, in air, food and water, loads the recognition and assessment functions of our immune systems. It is a loading they would do much better without. One sign of the significance of this loading is the growth of allergic responses. These are not infections, although allergic reactions can be precipitated by the effects of pathogens. The vast increase in allergic problems today is one result of contamination by artificial chemical molecules of every part of our global environment. From the environment they end up inside us, causing immune memory overload. The most common response to such overload is an allergic reaction. But even if this does not occur, our immune systems will be compromised in other ways. Pollution of any sort is a fundamental aid to disease.

After air, food and water, the most significant disease vector is other people. Infected people become sources of more infectious organisms, which are returned to the fundamental vectors. Infected people aid the momentum of the spread of the disease. The closer people are to other people the easier it is for airborne infections to spread. Measles, for example, cannot survive in communities where the birth-rate drops below 10,000 per year. If you were given the problem of spreading diseases, modern cities with mass transport, modern offices with air conditioning and large stores would be essential ingredients for success.

Some diseases spread by bodily contact: the close contact diseases. These range from fungus infections spread by skin contact, to sexually transmitted disease, which requires the exchange of contaminated fluids between one body and another.

It is because these routes are so basic to our survival that our protagonists have also found them suitable for their success. Peripheral vectors involve a large element of chance, or bad luck.

8

Wounds and injuries involve chance. If we are injured, and our skin torn or ruptured, any pathogen in the air has immediate and almost unhindered access to our inner processes. Before our understanding of disease mechanisms, even the most trivial wound could have been fatal. This was true in the fairly recent past, aided by our misunderstanding of the ways our bodies fought infections. During the First World War attempts at antisepsis frequently had more adverse effects on natural immune functions than on infections. The result of excessive sterilization of open wounds was that more of those treated tended to die than those who were not. The best treatment was to change clean dressings frequently; these allowed the immune system to deal with the infection, stopped further invasions, and removed the expelled debris before it became a source of re-infection. As a young doctor, Alexander Fleming, who subsequently discovered penicillin, was involved in the observations which revealed this principle; no doubt its implications deeply impressed him. It was only with the coming of the sulphonamide drugs in the 1930s, and penicillin in the 1940s, that we had effective means of aiding the immune system in its battle against established internal infections.

Infections are also spread by penetrating wounds from animals and plants. Rabies is the best-known example of disease transmitted via a wound from an animal. The organism passes from the saliva of the infected animal into the blood of the bitten person. Being pricked by a thorn can also transmit disease. Sleeping Beauty and Snow White were probably victims of tetanus bacteria, rather than wicked witches. Such bacteria produce an extremely toxic substance which induces paralysis; this can persist for some time before the body is overwhelmed.

Blood-eating insects, such as mosquitoes and fleas, also spread disease. Before such insects start feeding they usually inject their victim with fluid which will prevent the blood clotting. If the insect has previously dined on an infected victim, it will have picked up some of the infectious organisms, or their eggs, with its meal. Although not all infections drawn into insects are passed on, in some cases they will multiply within the insect, so that the next dinner gets a super dose with the anticoagulant. In other cases, they may be passed on incidentally.

Pathogens

The perspective of health developed in this book is based on a holistic philosophy. This means that, in addition to considering the harm caused by pathogens, we will also look at any useful place our enemies may have in the overall scheme of things. It is very limiting, and ultimately self-defeating, to view those things which attack us only in terms of disease. A holistic view seeks to enhance *all* life, even if some of its forms have to be avoided or kept in their place.

Viruses are tough and adaptable. They are fascinating creatures which exist on the border between matter and life. The best way to envisage them is as a strand of genetic material encapsulated in a tough coating – a life-form in a spaceship. Some can lie around almost indefinitely, enduring heat and cold, drought or flood, to awaken when they come into contact with a potential host. To reproduce, viruses have to get inside the cells of a much more complex compatible plant or animal. Once inside, they set about perverting the cell's genetic codes. Instead of doing what it should, the cell reproduces more of the virus. Eventually the cell collapses from exhaustion, and hordes of new viruses spread out to multiply by invading other cells. When this happens, you are infected; you will go down with 'flu or measles or whatever illness the virus causes.

Your viruses will be passed on to others. The growing population in your body will spill out into our shared global environment. They will add to the virus numbers in the disease's specific vector; by breathing out clouds of them into the air, or into food and drink; by passing them on by bodily contact; by releasing them into the environment in bodily wastes; or by feeding them to intermediate insect hosts such as mosquitoes.

Viruses are everywhere. They float in the air we breathe and the water we drink. They are a natural and constant part of the microscopic background to life. Frequently they will not affect us, because we have acquired immunity to them. Some remain in our bodies in a form of coexistence, as with the herpes virus which causes chicken pox (*Varicella zoster*), which will flare up when immunity, usually gained in childhood, has decreased sufficiently. In middle age this is experienced as an attack of shingles, which dies down once immunity is re-established.

Every now and then a new strain of a common virus will emerge and sweep around the world. When this happens we are reminded of the potential danger of virus infections; 'flu can be a killer, particularly of the very young and the old or enfeebled. New strains arise because of the ability of many viruses to change the structure of their protective coating. It is the molecular shape of this coat that our immune systems identify; by changing it viruses become immune to us. The AIDS virus seems extremely adept at changing its structure.

We frequently behave as if evolution stopped once Darwin had initiated the debate upon it. Unfortunately this is not so; very rarely a new type of pathogen will emerge. Sometimes an established infection of another species will adapt to survive within us, or evolution will throw up a new entity. As AIDS tragically illustrates, evolution continues in the microsphere. We will always have to confront the possibility of the appearance of entirely new types of disease for which we have no specific answers.

Viruses are remnants from the very beginning of life on Earth. They have evolved one step beyond the first replicating molecules in the primeval probiotic soup to have a protective coat around their active genetic material.

The next stage in the broad evolution of life was the formation of the cell, the basic structure upon which all subsequent life-forms have been built. Cells are basically sophisticated replicating molecules, genes, inside their own protective environment. Originally all such environments were mobile, but, like most mobile homes, cells soon discovered the advantages of congregating in groups. The viruses adapted to this innovation by learning to penetrate the cellular environment. Once inside, the ancient competition to reproduce by stealing resources or perverting processes is much as it was those many thousands of millions of years ago at the dawn of life. The odds against viruses being able to adapt in this way must have been astronomical. It is an indication of their high survival capacity which we overlook at our cost.

Bacteria are more complex. These ubiquitous microbes are single-cell organisms which reproduce by dividing into two. Their great talent is as chemical engineers; they take in substances through their cell membranes from the environment and transform them into useful products. Their purpose is to feed so that they may grow and reproduce. The activity of bacteria in fulfilling this basic aim makes all other life possible.

Every part of the planetry biosphere teems with bacteria. Plants depend upon them for their food in the soil, we depend upon plants to oxygenate the air and provide food. Bacteria are continually breaking down and recycling the basic molecular materials necessary for life. We may not like to acknowledge it, but our own digestive processes depend upon the activities of colonies of bacteria which live in our gut. They manufacture vitamin K, essential for blood clotting, and make some nutrients available to us that our digestive processes cannot produce. A course of antibiotics, particularly tetracycline, can cause weeks of bowel upset by killing too many of the goodies along with the baddies; things get back to normal when the goodies re-establish themselves. This illustrates both our open-ended commitment to our shared environment, and our intimate dependence on the talents of bacteria.

Since Louis Pasteur confirmed the existence of the bacterial microsphere, the germ theory of disease and our overreaction to it has been central to our concept of illness. Yet if we were to kill all known germs dead, we would rapidly follow them into extinction. Nevertheless it is true that not everything bacteria do is good, and their occupation of some environments can cause trouble. If this happens to be inside your body, the wrong bacteria in the wrong place, you may suffer from a bacterial infection. In dealing with bacteria and coexisting with them, understanding becomes crucial and a balanced approach essential.

Problem bacteria tend to pick specific parts of the body to inhabit. *Meningococcal* bacteria invade the brain, where they can cause meningitis; *tubercule* bacteria go for the lungs, and cause tuberculosis. Some can cause problems in many sites, such as *staphylococci*, which cause skin boils, sore throats, blood poisoning, or osteomyelitis if they get into bones.

Like viruses, many bacteria can go into a dormant state where they are highly resistant to unfavourable conditions. Once they find a favourable environment they reproduce rapidly; many can double their population every fifteen minutes. At this rate, one bacterium can become sixteen million in only six hours, and thirty-two million fifteen minutes later. This doubling of numbers in a fixed time is called exponential growth; it is characteristic of many life processes. It explains how particularly virulent bacteria can overwhelm us so quickly. Some victims of the Black Death 'woke well at dawn, to be dead by noon', as one observer noted.

Slightly more sophisticated than bacteria are the life-forms broadly classified as *flagellates*, *protozoa* and *amoebae*. These are all microscopic life-forms and some live parasitically in humans. They cause conditions such as vaginal trichomonas, diarrhoea and malaria. For most practical purposes we may think of them as bacteria.

The fungi which infect our bodies mainly grow on our skin and mucous membranes; they like areas which are frequently damp. Fungi as a whole come in a range of shapes and sizes. We are all familiar with edible mushrooms and poisonous toadstools; some fungi are large, some microscopically small, some invisible and others very colourful. Fungi and moulds are traditionally associated with death and decay. Although they are plants, fungi have no chlorophyll, the green substance which allows other plants to manufacture food by photosynthesis; because of this fungi live by feeding on ready-made organic matter.

Some of the smaller fungi give us useful products. Penicillin is produced by a mould, as in blue cheese, and the yeast sub-group is active in everything from alcohol to our daily bread. Much fungal activity complements the useful work done by bacteria in recycling waste. It is fungal activity which breaks up fallen leaves and converts them to the fertile fine-textured leaf mould found on forest floors. As we may know to our cost, it is also fungal activity which breaks up dead wood.

Fungi also live parasitically on plants and animals. If you are their chosen diet of ready-made organic matter, you may not feel too enthusiastic about this sort of activity. Fungi feed by excreting an enzyme on to the surface where they are growing; this digests the living matter, which is then absorbed by the fungus. This method of attack, and the immune system's counter-attack with toxic chemicals, gives you some idea why fungal infections such as athlete's foot and thrush are characteristically itchy.

The last creatures our immune systems tackle are worms. Worms are about halfway up the evolutionary ladder. In essence they are cells which have combined to form one tube inside another. Like bacteria and fungi, most worms live industrious and very useful lives, existing as free-living agents in earth and water. Unfortunately, some exist as parasites in both plants and animals. Those we are concerned with are almost microscopic, and around a hundred species are parasitic in humans. Like bacteria, they can invade almost every organ of the body, and the preferred sites of particular species produce specific disease conditions in much the same way as bacteria produce disease.

Serious worm problems are more common in tropical and sub-tropical regions. In these areas one species, the hookworm, causes untold misery and, indirectly, the deaths of millions. Infected children tend to be both physically and mentally retarded, contributing to the cycle of poverty and deprivation upon which the worm depends. The hookworm problem could be solved very simply by two measures: wearing shoes and digging deep holes to dispose of human excreta. Both measures depend, like most measures which create health, upon minor amounts of money combined with major changes in the attitudes of the potential victims.

Temperate zone worm problems are rarely fatal. The most common are infestations of the digestive tract, which are easily dealt with by poisoning the worms. Those worms which can cause us most damage are those for whom we are *accidental* hosts. The best known is the trichina worm (*Trichinella spiralis*) which normally lives in pigs and rats. Humans become infected by eating pork containing the larval stage of the worm. The answer to trichina worms is more simple than to hookworms; make sure all pork is well cooked. Fortunately infections with trichina are fairly rare, as the rat–pig part of their life-cycle has become progressively disrupted.

Those are the four main groups of living organisms with which our immune system deals. In addition, it tackles a wide variety of other foreign bodies which enter our bodies. These are either metabolized (that is, broken down for disposal) or moved to the surface to be expelled or lost with replaceable tissues.

Toxins

The *Concise Oxford Dictionary* defines a toxin as a 'poison especially of animal or vegetable origin; poison formed in body by pathogenic organism'.

13

Definitions change with time; a toxin was originally a substance used to poison Greek arrows. Today we need to extend the meaning of toxin, in the sense of a poison, to any substance our bodies have difficulty dealing with. Such difficulty will result in some form of toxic reaction.

Many substances can have adverse effects on the response of our immune system. The problem is that it is not possible to draw up a list of these substances, mark them 'dangerous' and thus solve the problem. Their effects in a population will form a continuum; individual differences will be reflected in varying responses according to differing metabolic characteristics. Some substances are unambiguously dangerous. The heavy metals, such as lead and cadmium, which circulate as pollutants in the environment, are known to aid disease in a variety of ways.

The problem arises with many of the 40,000 or so artificial molecules now circulating in the environment. These are made by the chemical industry and turned into a wide variety of products, from plastics to food additives. Every area of our life involves such substances; it is difficult to avoid them. These entirely artificial molecules complement the damage done by natural poisons. We evolved to live with some of these natural substances, but our manipulation of many aspects of our environment means that we are now exposed to grossly unnatural amounts of them. Nitrate fertilizers, which pollute water courses and turn into toxic nitrites, are an increasingly common example.

While each of the substances we produce and use is assessed as 'safe' (except for those used as poisons, in agriculture and so on), the effect of many such substances acting together is rarely assessed. Yet this is exactly the problem we expect our immune systems to tackle. The immune system is the gate-keeper of access to our bodies at many levels. It has to deal with all the chemicals we breathe, eat and drink in the modern world. While an expert may say that a particular substance, be it food additive, solvent or cleanser, is safe on its own, it would be foolish to claim that a random mixture of ten, or a hundred, or a thousand of them in varying proportions is safe *beyond doubt*.

The problem of toxins is further complicated by variations in individual response. Each of us will respond differently to a different dose and range of such substances. Some might get spots, others develop allergies, others find their immune system compromised when required to fight off infection. While hard proof of damage from such a wide-ranging source of usually low-level pollution is unattainable, the association is strong enough for many to be in no doubt. Many modern chemical industry products amount to low-level poisons, and our bodies treat them as such. We use up valuable capacity dealing with this self-imposed burden.

By now you may be feeling a little uncomfortable, wondering which part of your body battlefield is going to cave in first. Be reassured. Your immune system is running a vast protective enterprise non-stop, night and day, on your behalf.

Immune Action

With all the possible vectors for disease into our bodies, it is inevitable that some pathogens will get through and our immune systems will swing into action against them. To protect us these systems have to assess *everything* which enters our bodies. There are no exceptions. It does not matter whether they are some of the life-forms discussed above, food and drink, or substances polluting our environment.

At some point decisions are taken in our body on the molecules of everything we ingest. This process of assessment is much more complex than asking, 'Friend or foe?' The first stage is to decide if the substance is 'self', a part of our body or its constituents, or 'non-self', something from outside. If non-self, the substance – whether protein coating on a virus, cell structure of a bacterium, molecules of food we are eating, or pollen or pollution we are breathing – has to be checked against libraries of records. These are believed to be stored in the crystalline structure of mast cells. These specialized cells are found in every part of our bodies, particularly at joints and junctions between different sorts of cells, and they are especially numerous on membranes which are open to the environment. If the shape of an incoming molecular structure matches one on record, the response will be either *known-harmless*, in which case nothing happens; or *known-harmful*, when it will be marked for destruction by the immune system. Chapter 3 will explain how this is done.

The last category of assessment, *not-known*, is the one which is of most interest. Our response can be complex and varied, or there may be no response at all. Responses to the same substance will vary from individual to individual, and will be modified by things which are inhibiting or compromising our immune systems, and the inherent efficiency of those systems. The efficiency of response will depend in turn on many factors. In malnourished

15

populations measles can produce epidemics with very high rates of fatality; among the very old and very young common viruses like influenza cause death. Healthier people tend to resist all infections better than those who are feeble or debilitated.

The final problem our immune system deals with is cancer. Our bodies are producing faulty, potentially cancerous, cells all the time. These are taken apart and their components recycled by the immune system. Cancer wins when malignant cells are produced faster than the system can dispose of them, or when part of the mutation includes resistance by the cancerous cells to the destructive efforts of the immune system.

Cancer is a complex problem. Faulty cells can be produced for many reasons, from the influence of some viruses to chemical or radiological disruption. These cells reproduce at abnormal rates, creating the colonies of faulty cells we know as cancers. But like many things which present themselves as complex and apparently insoluble, there is frequently an underlying simplicity which holds the key to solution. With cancer it is this: 80 per cent of the cancers we suffer are avoidable. Not curable by early detection, but avoidable altogether. Until we come to our senses, and cease to create conditions which spread this burden of suffering and death, the only realistic option is to do everything we can to avoid known carcinogens (substances which cause cancers) and adopt a way of living which helps our immune system keep on top.

The same dual approach is the only answer for the new infections. We can avoid them by disrupting their approach vectors and making sure our systems resist any that get through. This is the only answer for potentially fatal conditions such as AIDS, Rift Valley fever, Legionnaires' disease, and any other new infection. With these conditions we may not be aware of the points of possible infection, and many of the vectors may be impossible to control or beyond our power to influence. The only safe option is to take whatever avoiding action we can and maximize immunity. This option may prove vital.

The same is true of allergic reactions. These are caused by mistakes made by our immune systems. Most food allergies appear to be quite simple — sufferers become allergic to a particular food. But why does this happen, when the food is very common, like grains or milk, and they have probably been eating it for years? It is either because their immune system is overloaded in some area and making a mistake, or because it is reacting to process residues or additives in the food rather than to the food itself.

Allergic reactions such as hay fever occur when our mast cells react strongly to substances they classify incorrectly. They react by degranulating, a kamikaze attack on the intruder provoked by mistaken identity. Degranulating releases a potent chemical barrage, including histamines, designed to kill the intruder. Fortunately, allergic reactions are usually experienced as low-level responses to environmental pollutants. Those substances which the body may treat as toxic, drawn from any of the 40,000 or so artificial chemicals now circulating in our environment, may not be the direct cause of problems, but by overloading our assessment systems, they cause malfunctions in the immune records.

Hay fever is a good example of the effects of this overload. Hay fever was unknown before the industrial revolution; now between 10 and 20 per cent of the population of every industrial nation suffer, and the number of victims increases every year. Many believe that pollen *causes* hay fever. However, since we evolved through millions of years in close proximity to it, blaming pollen for the explosion of hay fever over the last two hundred years is illogical. The truth is that these organic particles trigger the reaction we know as hay fever. The triggering substance is mis-identified by the overloaded system, and in desperation mast cells degranulate releasing histamine and other chemical agents, which cause sneezing, snuffling and swelling.

The trouble is that once our systems have learned to produce allergic reactions they tend to take this option more frequently. Once triggered by one substance, we become sensitized to others, and become more prone to allergies of all sorts as our immune systems seek to shed their overload.

Not all overloads result in allergic reactions. The more usual effect is a general lowering of resistance to infections. Looking at the population at large, subjected as it is to increasing stress and pollution, this is exactly the picture we observe. Virus infections appear to be enjoying a boom. While AIDS is the most serious example, surveys report that other conditions, which are life-limiting rather than life-threatening, are also on the increase.

Boosting Immunity

Let us state the basic requirements of a strategy for health. It will be necessary to shed some worn-out attitudes. The medieval view that those who succumbed to infectious disease did so through bad luck, or the adverse expression of divine opinion, lingers on today. Our attitudes to disease can influence its effects. The idea that disease has any direct link with morality should be rejected. Pathogens, like humans, are natural phenomena subject to natural laws.

We have to be aware of the vectors diseases occupy on the routes into our bodies. Avoiding, disrupting or closing these is our first line of defence, analogous to intelligence and sabotage in warfare. The lessons of hygiene, care with food and uncontaminated water are as relevant today as they have ever been. But the world is a more complex place than the one in which these truths were discovered. Today we generate pollution in the name of cleanliness, malnutrition in the name of convenience, and health hazards in the name of commercial freedom.

In our pressurized world it cannot be denied that luck, in the sense of being in the wrong place at the wrong time, plays a part in all the hazards of modern life. And that the variations in genetic make-up, together with ante- and post-natal influences, will predispose some more than others to particular disease risks. But it is equally undeniable that we can do much to improve our chances of avoiding trouble.

We must accept that the infectious pathogens with which we are dealing are highly adaptable survivors. They inhabited the Earth for countless millennia before us, and show no sign of losing their adaptability or grip on life. Indeed, rather the opposite is true; if AIDS is an isolated example of a new type of infectious organism we face a disaster; if it is the first of many similar infections the future for humanity could be bleak.

Our most important strategy for health begins with understanding this truth: we can expect no weakness or surrender from our adversaries. The only option is to improve our strength. By strengthening our immune system, working with it rather than damaging it through ignorance or neglect, we can increase our resistance to a wide range of illnesses, minor and serious, commonplace and rare.

Much of the apparently unimportant detail of the way we live imposes needless stress on our immune system, leaving us 'immune compromised' as the jargon puts it, or in plain language, potential victims. We can exercise choice and remove this burden, allowing our immune system to function more efficiently, dealing with the things it was designed to tackle.

Infections, allergies and cancers can all result from immune-system failure.

18

We can radically reduce the risk from all these problems by appropriate action. The next chapter outlines the essentials for an instant improvement of immunity function.

2

An Instant Improvement

Your immunity can be instantly improved by adopting the following habits:
* Eating enough good food
* Avoiding pollution – particularly tobacco smoke
* Getting regular strenuous physical activity
* Resting adequately
* Feeling positive about yourself

The order does not matter; each is important, although the relevance of specific items to any particular individual will vary. Nor is there any cross-compensation; even if you are physically active, you cannot carry on smoking. Similarly, even if you eat as we recommend, you cannot maintain high immunity without adequate sleep.

The best way to achieve the necessary changes in your lifestyle is to read this chapter with a notebook. As we deal with each topic, note how far you are from the ideal. You will then be able to decide which is your weakest area; you should start initiating change here, so that eventually all areas match the ideal as far as is possible.

Do not underestimate the task. Most people find it extremely difficult to change their behaviour patterns. Even when we know it is essential that we do so, it can still take time, consistent effort and persistence. We are held on our old unsatisfactory course by unconscious attitudes which are hard to

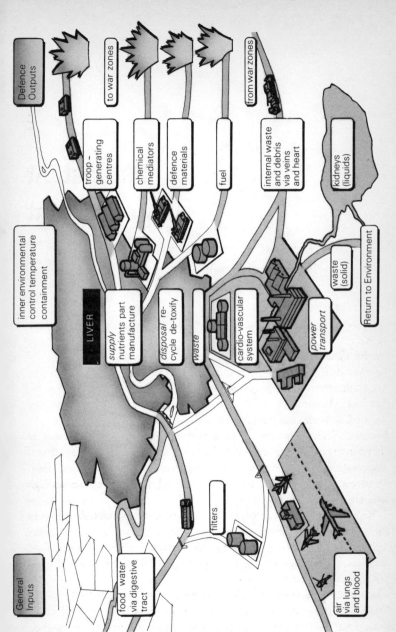

Figure 3

change. Normally we rely on them to guide us correctly without the need to think everything out every time we have to make a choice. But when we have been given the wrong set of mental attitudes, change is essential. Those who can achieve a new mindset in the light of new circumstances are those who can adapt; they tend to be the survivors in situations where the old wisdom no longer applies.

One mechanism our mind employs to preserve old attitudes is *cerebration*. Cerebration is the creation of an internal belief which does not match the outward expression. Armchair enthusiasts are cerebrators; they read about gardening or sport or watch it on TV, and imagine they perform the activities they read about or watch. Surveys have shown that many more people say they play tennis when Wimbledon is on TV than at other times of the year. The mind acknowledges the belief that something is good for us, but because achieving it requires a change of attitude the mind short-circuits. It just sends back DONE, instead of doing it. Anyone trying to change their lifestyle should be aware of this cop-out cover-up; make sure you really do what you believe you should do.

22

Primary Objective

Each of the five factors listed above is essential for the achievement of a primary objective which will underwrite the activity of your whole immune system. This is to improve your metabolic efficiency. You cannot improve your natural immunity without doing this; metabolic efficiency is the equivalent of economic and industrial efficiency in war.

Look at Figure 3. On the left are General Inputs, the necessities we have to draw from our shared global environment: food, water and air. These are taken into our bodies via lungs and the digestive tract. As we saw in the previous chapter, these open routes are also used by pathogens and toxins to gain access. The products of these inputs, in their various forms, eventually arrive in the liver. The liver is the centre of the body's industrial area.

Powering the system, and providing transport for the body's materials, is the heart. The complex cardio-vascular system picks up oxygen from the lungs, and delivers it around the body and to the liver; it also carries nutrients from the digestive tract to the liver, and carries products from the liver around the body. In addition it picks up waste and transports it for disposal, mainly to the liver and kidneys.

The heart is at the centre of a complex multi-functional system, connected with all other parts of our bodies. Our diagram only shows the main lines relevant to its partnership with the liver, but it is important to realize that the overall efficiency of the cardio-vascular system depends upon the blood vessels. If they have not been fully developed, or have become clogged or damaged, then the immune system will not get the troops and materials it needs, particularly in distant parts of the body.

On the right we have the Defence Outputs. These will be dealt with in detail later. Notice that, with the exception of oxygen, all the basic raw materials needed for the war against pathogens originate in the liver. In addition to supplying battle and building needs, it also regulates much of what goes on around our bodies. Both heart and liver are basic to our survival, and the quality of the service we get from them is crucial to immunity.

That is not to say they are the only factors involved in our constant battle; many others play vital parts. But without the liver the others are useless. Nations at war like to bomb each other's factories because without factories and power the armies will grind to a halt; those better supplied will tend to win. It is just the same in our bodies; our general objective is to ensure that the immune system has the better supplied troops.

Liver Function

A good way to visualize the liver is as a vast marshalling yard, with thousands of factories along the incoming and outgoing lines, with roads running across the tracks connecting different lines of factories, with power and communication lines linking every unit to all the others. Molecular trains are constantly arriving, being broken down and modified, and shipped out again to perform various functions around the body. The nervous system provides signals, sensors and access to the computer of our brain.

Digested food is carried directly into the liver by the hepatic portal vein, the main route into the marshalling yard. In addition to nutrients the blood will be carrying a wide range of other substances, some of them highly undesirable. The liver metabolizes – that is, breaks down for recycling or waste – almost everything which enters it. This will include everything which enters, or is produced by, our body. It will range from digested food to cancer cells and cellular debris; viruses and bacteria and their waste and

23

by-products; hormones, both self-produced and imposed; drugs and toxins. It deals with fat being recycled for energy. With our kidneys it keeps the constituents of our blood in balance.

In the liver, blood, rich in digestive products and the assortment of other things it carries, circulates through six-sided 'liver lobules'. The liver is made up of these lobules, each one similar to all the others, yet each a highly sophisticated organ in its own right. The lobules are the factories in the marshalling yard, where the complicated processes of biotransformation take place.

With all this processing going on, there is inevitably a lot of waste. Waste disposal is important because if the system cannot cope it will be overwhelmed and fail. The usual disposal route is back into the blood, and out via our kidneys into the shared environment once more. Substances that take this route have first to be made water soluble. Those that cannot be dissolved in water are dissolved in fat. Thence they are carried in the bile, which is secreted into the bile duct, and back into the digestive tract. If they take the hint these substances are eliminated as semi-solid waste to the environment.

24

Unfortunately the semi-solid waste system is not very efficient. To save effort and resources, the endlessly busy liver recycles bile, only losing small amounts with waste; inevitably some of the garbage gets recycled as well. This is the untidy end of the marshalling yard. There is some advantage in this disorder; the levels of some substances can be kept more or less constant, thus saving efforts for other systems. Within the body the dangers of over-zealous housekeeping are recognized; economy of effort is combined with achieving a multiplicity of ends. The danger of this admirable regime is that undesirable and unwanted substances also get left behind, and they can build up in the system if it is not run as intended.

Because metabolism is complicated, there are many subroutines for dealing with a wide range of problems, including the build up of wastes. Frequently there will be options, and such decisions will be influenced by other factors affecting the metabolism. The final result of some of these options may not be what we consider desirable. Some may hinder our immune system, or ultimately produce diseases, such as cardio-vascular conditions or diabetes, which have their roots in metabolic problems.

One common subroutine, particularly for women, is concerned with the manufacture of fat. When confronted by a substance it considers too toxic to handle, the liver refuses to metabolize it. Instead it will manufacture fat in which it will store the substance on the body until 'later'. This indicates gross overload; you need your liver to do more constructive things than make fat. The answer to liver overload resulting from pollution and toxic accumulation is simple: you have to exclude as many such pollutants and poisons as possible from your general inputs.

The object of achieving maximum metabolic efficiency is to ensure a rapid response when your body comes under attack. At these times it will need more of the outputs on the right-hand side of the diagram: materials to generate troops, chemical mediators, defence materials, and fuel. To avoid going down with infections, it is essential that all necessities for immune-system battles are produced as quickly and efficiently as possible. Having to deal with imposed overloads as a matter of routine severely limits this capacity.

The liver also exerts control over the battle zones in the body (Inner Environment Control, see Figure 3). It does this by responding to feedback from infected sites. The subtle changes the liver can induce are all designed to help the front-line immunity troops to deal with the enemy; sometimes, when the battle is widespread, the effects are not so subtle, as when we run a very high temperature. These changes can be crucial in some battles, so as a general principle we should hinder them as little as possible.

Metabolic efficiency, maximum liver and heart capacity, and minimum avoidable overload, are essential prerequisites for improving your immunity. These are the firm foundation upon which all health is built, and as such are indispensable. In their absence we are left treating one emergent condition after another, never fully well, a situation which has become the norm in our society.

Improvements

Eating and Drinking

Eating and drinking *enough* of the right sort of things is vital for health. This is a basic and unavoidable fact. Wrong choices or bad habits in nutritional input are practically impossible to correct by other means. It is important that we feed ourselves well and adequately.

Ideally, you should eat organically produced food, and filter your tap water, or drink bottled mineral water. Excessive and impossible? Twenty years ago most people would have thought so; ten years ago you might have been thought a little odd. Today it is the only way to ensure that what you are eating and drinking are not harming you. In changing over to this regime you will be joining a sizeable minority who have already done so.

If you also follow the traditional recommendation of dietitians and eat a well-balanced diet, you will have little if any of the multitude of problems which confront people on the modern processed and de-natured diet. For most people well-balanced means eating more fresh vegetables, particularly greens and salads, raw rather than cooked; more fish and other seafoods; more fruit, and more nuts, seeds and grains.

There are three good food rules which everyone should bear in mind:

1) Organic is best; always go for the best
It may cost more, but it is worth it. Remember, you are paying twice the shop price for most foods through tax subsidies to farmers and producers (not to mention EEC intervention costs to store all the contaminated food nobody eats). Most organic growers are small and local, and do not get this assistance.

2) Good food is food which will go bad
You should buy fresh food and eat it at its best. If its best lasts a long time, it is usually because it has been treated with preservatives. The exceptions are dried beans, grains and fruits; these are normally re-hydrated when they can once more go bad easily. Vegetables, such as onions, potatoes, swedes, carrots, etc., are usually sprayed with anti-fungals and hormones to stop them sprouting. Organic roots are not sprayed, so you may not have continuous supplies of everything you may want. The answer is to eat seasonally; go for what is being naturally produced at the time.

3) The best food is the least processed food
Wholefoods are foods which have had none of their edible parts removed. They are obviously superior although they may not always be organic. For example, consider the many forms of rice sold in large supermarkets. There are various types of white and 'quick-cooking' rice; these have been polished, and their natural bran coating, which contains important B-group vitamins and minerals as well as protein, has been removed. Do not buy white rice. There will also be brown rice; this is complete with its bran coat and has a reasonable level of nutrients, and is a type of wholefood. Finally, there is organic brown rice, which is highest in nutrients and the best and tastiest type you can get.

26

Wholefoods are generally darker in colour and rougher in texture. You can't usually cook light, fluffy and insubstantial dishes with wholefoods, but they have far more flavour, and they are what your body was designed to digest.

Why is this care with food and drink necessary? A casual observer might imagine that we would have long ago solved any problems concerning nutrition. In fact, the opposite is nearer the truth. Most people in the West do not eat enough nutritious food. Deficiencies of vitamins and minerals are endemic. From the health point of view most of the food on sale in the average high street is extremely suspect, some downright harmful. It would only require a small supermarket basket to collect those items which are above any suspicion.

Over the last forty years there has been a revolution in the food industry. Since the end of the War – when the nation had to feed itself well to survive – wholesome, traditional produce has been replaced by factory-farmed and processed products. The new products' relationship with wholesome nature is largely confined to the folksy picture printed on the pack to entice the consumer. There is a continuing battle to force manufacturers to disclose on the label exactly what the pack contains, but this misses much of the point; what such foods *lack* is equally important.

Modern farming uses three basic chemicals in fertilizers (nitrate, potassium and phosphate). These produce large plants but do not replace the other nutrients which plants take from soil. Worse, they can inhibit the uptake of vital nutrients into plants. The longer chemical farming continues, the larger the impoverished crop and the greater the impoverishment of the soil. So we create a cycle of larger but more harmful harvests. Subsequent processing of food further decreases the micronutrient content. As if this were not bad enough, chemical additives are then used to increase non-nutritional properties, such as shelf life, colour and profitability. The end product is a cocktail with little to recommend it.

It has taken a long time for us to accept that just because a product is for sale does not mean it is safe or good for us. Recent concern over food additives only scratches the surface of the problem. Ordinary food contains a wide variety of pesticide and drug residues – pesticides from the almost continuous spraying of crops and drug residues from the hormones and antibiotics without which the unnatural lifestyle of the animals we eat would be impossible. Even fish from the sea bring back to our plates the residues of pesticides sprayed long ago on to the land. Not so slowly, but very surely, we are poisoning our shared global environment, all its produce and ourselves.

We accept that each of the substances involved in modern food production may be safe in low concentrations for the majority of people. We also accept that many people will be able to cope for some time on a diet which contains many such substances. But we can only describe as very fortunate those who have bodies efficient enough to cope, day after day, with the assault the modern food industry delivers.

The fact is that as this assault grows in intensity and complexity fewer people are able to cope with it. As the progressive industrialization of food continues, our metabolism is forced to work harder. Each new artificial molecule has to be assessed and dealt with by systems which are finely tuned to deal with the range of substances they encountered during our evolution. It may be just polytetrafluroethylene to you, but to your immune system it could be an insurmountable puzzle. Our evolutionary development was very slow; we simply cannot keep up with what is happening today.

We are at the top of many food chains. As each level, from bacteria upwards, concentrates these artificial chemicals, we become the recipients of such substances. We adulterate our food at every level, from birth or synthesis, to table. It is no exaggeration to say that much of the chronic disease and the groundswell of malaise which affects us, together with our increasing susceptibility to allergies, cancers and infections, can be traced back to the way we feed ourselves.

Buying organic food will require deliberate effort. Some supermarkets are beginning to stock some lines, but they are the exception. Check out your local market; many growers who come in one or two days a week will be glad to discuss their methods and produce with you. Only some of the goods in your local wholefood shop will be organically produced; always check the labels. Paradoxically, city dwellers will find it fairly easy, as many new small shops are opening up to supply the increasing demand. Look for the following marks to be absolutely sure that what you are buying is organically produced:

Soil Association   *Bio-Dynamic Agricultural*   *Organic Farmers &*
                        Association   *Growers*

Of course you could grow your own. Even in the city you can sprout beans and seeds for fresh salads all the year round. If you have a small garden, producing organic vegetables can be very rewarding; use them to supplement freezing and bulk buying of staple foods such as grains.

Twentieth-century women are obsessed by dieting. Mothers discuss at what age they should start their daughters on diets. In a saner future, dieting will be seen as the mass insanity of our age. It does not keep you slim and it is bad for your health, yet the belief that by suffering self-imposed famine the salvation of slimness will result is one of the most deeply entrenched errors of our current mindset. The most important step towards improving your immunity and creating health is to change outdated attitudes; changing the current erroneous attitude to dieting is a prime example.

To maximize your immunity you *must* supply your body with all the raw materials it needs to work efficiently. Imposing false conditions of famine does not do this. Eating enough of the right sorts of food will *not* make you fat, provided you are living a healthy lifestyle. Following all the recommendations in this chapter should ensure that you are doing this.

A wholefood diet which supplies sufficient nutrients to meet the needs of an average woman will deliver at least 2,000 calories per day; a man may need 3,000 or more. This represents a considerable bulk of food; you may have to get accustomed to larger portions and fuller plates.

How do you know when you are eating enough? It is very simple; you are eating enough when you feel hungry before eating and satisfied (not bloated) after your meals. If you never feel hungry, you may be suffering from malnutrition; zinc deficiency, a common result of a processed food diet, distorts or suppresses appetite.

We should all have some surface fat on our bodies. Not a lot, but enough to act as a buffer for energy demands and a metabolic reservoir. When you are established on a nutritionally adequate diet and you have an active lifestyle, you will be able to respond positively to body messages such as hunger without worrying about getting unhealthily fat.

Eating for maximum immunity means adopting a diet rich in the following foods:

Seafood, especially herring, eels, salmon and seaweed. Avoid shallow-water shellfish and crustacea, which concentrate pollutants.

Nuts, especially almonds, cashews, brazils and sunflower seeds, preferably raw.

Fresh yellow-fleshed fruit, especially apricots, peaches, mango, cantaloupe melon; eat citrus fruit with meals to enhance mineral absorption.

Organically produced liver. Liver concentrates both nutrients and toxins, which means that while it is very rich in nutrients, it can be highly polluted if the animal did not have an organic diet.

Dark green vegetables, especially watercress, parsley, peppers, broccoli; also lettuce, cabbage and sprouts.

Wheat-germ and whole-wheat products. *Avoid* adding bran to food; this is unnecessary with a wholefood diet, and will reduce uptake of nutrients from the gut.

Peas, beans, lentils and peanuts.

Free-range eggs. Egg white should be always be cooked. It is probably unwise to have more than eight eggs per week.

Just as food should be selected with care, so should drink. Pure water is best; regrettably, this is not what most of us can expect to get from our kitchen taps. Bottled natural mineral waters are ideal. Pure fruit or vegetable juices and herb teas made with filtered water are also fine.

Coffee and tea should be drunk only in moderation. Go for small quantities and high quality. Soft drinks are a chemical minefield and should not even be considered.

Alcohol should generally be avoided, particularly by women with their relatively small livers. Do not drink alcohol more than three times a week, and keep your intake below three measures in any day. Alcohol has a wide range of damaging effects on the body, including reduced nutrient absorption and increased risk of many cancers. It puts a load on the liver which interferes with optimal function.

Alcoholic drinks are subject to the same product development as any other commodity and are increasingly adulterated with chemicals. Go for traditional types if you drink spirits – vodka and malt whiskies being the safest (drink them neat, or with water or fruit juice); if you like long drinks, go for real ale. 'Bitter', 'mild' and nearly all lagers are dubious concoctions.

Avoiding Pollution – Particularly Tobacco Smoke

We must be clear about what we mean by pollution. This is another area where our ideas and attitudes are way out of date. The pollution problem today is not that which the word usually conjures up in our minds – smoke, dust and foul smells. While this sort of pollution does still exist, today's problem centres on all those thousands of artificial chemicals, some actually used because they smell nice, which we release intentionally in millions of tons every year into the environment. In addition our environment is polluted by natural substances which are generated in quantities which overload the biosphere; it simply cannot cope with some of our excesses.

Behind this front line of purposeful pollution is a second wave: all the toxic substances produced when we try to dispose of waste such as plastics and process intermediaries, and of course, all the radioactive products of the nuclear industry. We have failed to acknowledge the health problems of modern industry, hoping that, like the acid smoke from power-stations, they will go 'away'. They do not: they end up adversely affecting our health.

Traditionally we have used our environment as a giant dustbin where everything we have not wanted or found too nasty to handle has been thrown. From our diagrams of disease routes you will appreciate that we are each intimately connected with our shared environment. In poisoning it we are poisoning ourselves. Even if we do not feel the effects of the toxins we are circulating, they will weaken us, making us more susceptible to disease.

One concentrated area of pollution is the food- and drink-processing industry. By choosing organic food you will be helping to cut this off at source. You can also use your purchasing power to reduce other sources of pollution and make sure your home is as pollution free as possible. To find out how many products you have which are polluting your home environment, go through the questionnaire in Appendix 1 – and beware of cerebration. You do *not* need these things!

You may have to adjust your ideas once more. Getting rid of sanitizers, fresheners, disinfectants and cleansers will *improve* your health. Sadly, you have to throw these things 'away'. Decide that this will be the last time you do this to our environment; do not buy any more of these products. When enough of us make the same decision, the manufacturers will give up.

Another form of pollution you should do your best to avoid is vehicle exhaust fumes. The cloud of toxins produced by British cars, with leaded fuel, is particularly nasty. Our inability to legislate against outmoded technology may reflect Britain's declining economy or perhaps our misplaced social priorities. Whatever, we tend to accept it without question. Especially puzzling are those joggers who seem to prefer main roads where they gulp in lungfuls of lead and carbon monoxide together with all the other combustion products. Perhaps their real intention is to be seen, rather than be

31

healthy. Even in central London it is possible to find relatively unpolluted places to run.

Lead, like most heavy metals, damages the immune system. We can pick it up not only from vehicle exhausts but also from our water supply. Tap water contains many metals and minerals, the range and concentration of pollutants depending on the locality. To avoid these hazards use a water purifier such as a Brita Jug.

Old-fashioned smoke should be avoided, more so today because it is likely to contain new-fashioned pollutants. Burning rubbish should become a criminal offence; the only way to dispose of many modern wastes is in incinerators under carefully controlled conditions. Better, of course, not to produce waste in the first place. Everyday plastics can produce very dangerous toxins when burnt on bonfires. *Never burn plastics*.

If you are considering moving out to the country, be very careful. While publicity has been given to leukaemia clusters around nuclear installations, little has been said about the generally increased mortality around chemical industry sites. You should also avoid sites surrounded by open fields of arable farmland, especially in eastern England. These are likely to be sprayed with biocides for around ten months of the year. The best choice may be the seaside, with prevailing onshore winds; western hills with minimal chemical spraying; or suburbia with minimal traffic and industry. Remember, everywhere in the environment we have created, we are in retreat; this situation is illustrated by the difficulty of choosing somewhere healthy to live, particularly for children.

Whatever commerce and industry are doing to us and our environment, many of us add injury to insult. It remains a fact that the worst pollution we inflict upon ourselves is tobacco smoke. There is no reason why any of us should be subjected to this lethal hazard.

The 200-plus toxins in tobacco smoke are inflicted on us for two reasons. Firstly, nicotine is a highly addictive drug. Indeed it is unique, being simultaneously a tranquillizer and a stimulant. Those addicted have to treat their habit as seriously as they would addiction to heroin – there is no halfway house, no shortcut – you have to give it up. Secondly tobacco is very profitable. The government makes a lot of money out of cigarette smokers, more than it spends on 'treating' them for the inevitable diseases which lead to the early death of addicts. According to a review in the *Guardian* (6 May 1980) of an unpublished government report, 'successive governments have conceded privately that although DHSS officials are keen on anti-smoking legislation, counter-arguments from the Treasury or Departments of Trade or Employment have always won the day'.

The facts of the harm caused by tobacco are stark. In Britain it is responsible for 270 deaths every day. Cigarette smokers put themselves and others at risk from lung cancer, bronchitis and other respiratory infections, heart and circulatory disease. They also suffer from increased risk of cancers of the liver, pancreas and cervix. Dealing with these conditions bleeds away time and resources from medical care in every country in the world. It is little wonder that over the past few decades three separate US Presidential Commissions have recommended an outright ban on tobacco on health grounds. Unfortunately such calls for action have been defeated by the numbers of addicts, the tax revenue and the power of the tobacco industry.

If you wanted to create a welcoming environment for airborne infections, smoking would be hard to beat. Stimulating the over-production of mucus in the air ways, while paralysing the cilia that the body depends upon to dispose of it, and damaging the surface immune cells, gives pathogens a free, if not clear, passage to the throat and lungs.

Smoking has serious primary and secondary effects in the liver. Those who smoke to avoid putting on weight are relying on nicotine to change the balance of enzyme activity in their liver. This, in turn, disrupts the work of the liver in producing the outputs our body needs. The imbalance leads to waste and malnutrition. The ability of cigarette smoke to alter the detoxification systems of the liver could account for the fact that smoking is associated with cancers in many parts of the body where smoke never goes.

For many of its crucial functions the liver requires a good supply of oxygen, and adequate oxygen is essential to immune functions throughout the body. This is transported by the blood, which picks it up in our lungs. In smokers, the oxygen-carrying capacity of the blood is blocked by carbon monoxide. The concentration of this poisonous gas in the bloodstream is directly proportional to the number of cigarettes smoked (or the amount of exhaust fumes breathed).

The bad effects of smoking are exacerbated by other pollutants. Rates for diseases associated with the habit increase when the victims are subject to the additional pollution of inner-city or industrial environments.

Regular Strenuous Physical Activity

We are intended to be active, energetic, very physical animals. Not all of the time, but we should be capable of behaving in this way when circumstances demand. Against our nature our culture produces overwhelming pressures which make us passive and sedentary. Many people never experience the power and exhilaration their bodies can generate. They have been conditioned to associate activity with pain, drudgery, embarrassment and inferiority. These attitudes are more errors to be junked on the way to health. If you deny the physical side of your being, you may find it fails you when you require a supreme effort from it.

Ideally, at least twice, but no more than four times each week, you should undertake activity which is sufficiently strenuous to keep you hot enough to sweat, and which continues for between twenty and thirty minutes. The point is to generate the internal heat which causes you to sweat. (Sweating in a sauna is not the same!) Running is ideal, but any activity which demands sustained output from your body will do as well. Stop–start activities, such as tennis or even football, are not ideal. Appendix 2 gives suggested activities.

Warning: You may not be fit enough to become healthy! If you are unaccustomed to physical activity, getting on in years, or if there is the slightest danger of heart trouble, you must be realistic. If you are over thirty and lead an average life, but *think* you are fit and at no risk, check yourself out first. If you are exhausted you should not add to your stress level with strenuous activity. Those who work to excess are exactly the types who think they can or should bounce out and emulate Daley Thompson. This is utterly wrong; such people are only pushing themselves into further dangerous imbalance. If you are in danger of succumbing to this inclination, go on to the next improvement section and learn to rest before you learn to exercise.

If you are past your prime, do not despair. You can regain fitness and become very healthy, but it will take longer. Little but often should be your maxim. And you must accept that while you may never reach the ideal, any progress will bring health benefits. Everyone starting on a fitness course should do *half* of what they believe themselves capable. A graduated system, such as the Royal Canadian Air Force programme, is suitable for anyone wishing to become fit.

From the point of view of boosting immunity, the purpose of such activity is to stimulate the liver and increase its capacity. In achieving this you will also improve your cardio-vascular condition, and generate increased physical competence.

Regular strenuous physical activity is the only way to stimulate the liver.

34

The liver stores energy as glycogen in each of its lobules. When sufficiently stimulated, under the influence of adrenalin it will discharge its glycogen stores, giving that stream of energy known as 'second wind'. This is the source of energy that allows the exhausted walker, when confronted by a bull, to sprint and leap the hedge to safety. This discharge will cause the liver to recharge itself, from fat or food, and increase its function and capacity.

There is a profound difference between men and women which we must take into account. Women have livers which are much smaller than those of men. Stone for stone of body weight, the female liver is around half the size of that of the male.

The implications of this are two-fold. Firstly, the female detoxification capacity is smaller; this is why women's livers more readily opt to dump pollutants into fat. Avoiding pollution is very important for women. Secondly, the female body fuels itself differently to that of the male. Without the large-capacity liver and the explosive energy it can produce, women initially take fuel more from current-account food, and then from that subcutaneous fat layer. Because of the different mode of output between male and female bodies, they should also have different patterns of input. In general, women should be largely vegetarian nibblers and men feasting carnivores. Of course, in specific cases the situation is not that clear-cut, but ignoring these basic physiological differences can lead to difficulties.

Because the liver is our deepest store of immediate energy, it is hard to call on it in normal circumstances. The body is very careful in its use of energy. For habitual movements it builds up local capacity in muscles, so that we can do light or accustomed work for hours together without significantly affecting our liver. Activity has to be sufficiently strenuous to convince the liver we are serious and overcome its resistance. This is sometimes felt as a pain on the right-hand side of the chest. Once it has turned on, you will experience a flow of energy that needs to be burned up. That is the effect to aim for with your exercise programme.

Do not become an exercise fanatic. If you suspect your body is fighting an infection, you must stop any strenuous activity, since it is precisely these circumstances for which you have been preparing. Keep mobile and active if it feels right, take walks in fresh air, or perform an activity which aids relaxation. Do not try to turn your liver on; let it deal with the infection. When you have recovered (a lot quicker than you used to!), then build up the activity gradually. You may feel your liver resisting – a persistent pain on the lower right of your chest – for a week or two. Clearing up war-zone debris and eliminating the last pockets or resistance can take time. Be patient – listen to what your body is telling you.

Rest Adequately

It is essential that we all get sufficient sleep and relaxation, so that we wake each day feeling refreshed and alert, looking forward to the challenges and experiences ahead.

When we are active our brain pushes all its system switches to GO. In this position we can run through a range of responses suitable to our needs and the demands of particular situations. In this state, repairs, maintenance and growth are held back; temporary holding actions are taken. When we are relaxing or asleep, the switches are progressively pushed the other way, to HOLD. In this state all the positive recuperative activities take over, so that next time demands are made we can meet them.

Without adequate recuperation we gradually wear ourselves down. Eventually exhaustion allows disease in one form or another to overwhelm the body's defences. We are after the opposite effect. Provided we are well fed and not over-taxing ourselves, in the process of recovering from effort the body will over-compensate and build in more capacity than previously existed. This is part of the natural process of adaptation; by adopting the recommendations in this chapter, you will be directing this adaptive ability to increase your immunity and general health.

A common problem today, which is at the root of much stress disease, is that our brain *anticipates* action which does not happen. We sit in high-stress occupations, or excited in front of the TV, with all switches at GO. Under these conditions our brain believes we should be physically active, and it sends out appropriate messages and hormones. If we do not follow through and burn off the adrenalin, we find it difficult to relax and hard to sleep. Under these circumstances some people become addicted to adrenalin. In this way our brains can induce a state of stress; we can stress ourselves by just sitting still, another reason why being active is so important.

There is nothing wrong with stress as such. The important thing to realize is that it is intended to be a transient state. It is a capacity we have to meet a particular need. Stress is harmful when it becomes a permanent way of life, as would having to jump hedges to escape from bulls all the time. Women who stress their metabolism by enforced malnutrition in the name of slimness are helping disease, not health. Macho men, who fight on through infection and exhaustion, continuing to work when they should be recovering, just prolong their illness. In doing so they help it spread to many more victims.

With activity to restore hormone balance and adequate rest, stress need not cause problems for heart or immunity. It must be a part of a personal equation which is in balance.

Listen to your body; forget duties, 'oughts', the demands of others, and watch ambitions that take you nearer the morgue than the boardroom. If you need rest, take it. If you cannot relax, seek a means that helps – music, yoga, a stroll, sex, whatever works for you. Above all make sure that you get enough old-fashioned deep recuperative sleep. The traditional seven or eight hours is about what the average person needs. This amount of sleep is associated with a longer life. Unless you are very unusual, six hours or less each night will undermine your resistance to disease.

Feel Positive about Yourself

It is important to feel confident about yourself, in responding to your needs and your relationships with others; to feel in control of your life and able to cope with whatever circumstances you may confront.

Warning: We are dealing with emotions. In all our other recommendations we can say 'this is good (organic food, activity, etc.), and this is bad (processed food, an inactive lifestyle, etc.)'; when dealing with feelings we move rapidly away from any pretence of objectivity. We have to deal in intangible reactions, such as hope and happiness, which only you experience. The best we can do is to describe desirable states; *how* the internal reaction which represents this state is produced will vary widely from one individual to another. We all know some people we simply do not understand.

Our emotional responses are wide ranging, and they can be very powerful. While we are concerned with positive feelings, there are also negative emotions. In this dichotomy we confront all the extremes of life: love and hate, good and evil, life and death. In terms of health, the emotions we feel about ourselves, and those we project to the outside world, have different but important effects on us. Because they represent two dimensions within the same sphere, we require two objectives in dealing with them – honesty and control.

Emotional honesty can be summed up by the phrase 'Know thyself'. The simplicity of this axiom is illusory since there are many hurdles to achieving self-knowledge to the point where we can totally accept ourselves.

So far all the recommendations we have made for improving immunity and health are common sense and logical because of the basic nature of humans. Yet the lifestyle they represent is not the norm for the majority of people; to accept them we have to dismantle current assumptions which are deeply ingrained in our minds, both intellectually and emotionally. What is true of your inclinations towards choices in lifestyle is also true of choices in perception of yourself. We are nurtured in symbiosis with our culture. Culture gives us the values and perceptions by which we conduct our lives; in turn we contribute to its extension. This process creates the continuity of life which we experience.

Our problem, as highly cultured beings, is that we can never be entirely sure whether an emotion is ours, or a reflection of our culture. These reflections may be responses produced because of what we feel is expected of us, or what we have learned, consciously or subconsciously, in society, or projected upon us by the myriad of media with which we surround ourselves. The net result is that in our self-perception we are subject to many influences outside ourselves.

The practical result of such influences is that many people are brought up to be dishonest about their feelings. Individual responses are sacrificed in favour of those required by socio-cultural behavioural models. We know the way we 'ought' to behave, or believe we ought to feel, but frequently what we actually feel deep inside is something else entirely. We may feel extreme rage, but because we have been conditioned to believe that we should be nice, we express something which is emotionally dishonest. We harm ourselves when we believe the dishonest reaction we have been taught to express is our emotional reality.

Much of the popular personal growth therapy of the last decades has been based on understanding this premise. Getting in touch with your personal emotional reality is important; unless you can differentiate between reality and reflection you have little hope of fulfilling those desirable but intangible values of life, such as happiness, joy and love.

Love is important because it is where we find our most fulfilling emotional experiences. But love is a state fraught with disillusionment and disappointment. Indeed it can be so troublesome that the ancient Greeks regarded it as a disease; young people in particular were sent away until they recovered. The problems associated with love may stem from the fact that we are trying to match two sets of reality and reflection, usually when the mirrors of perception are being shaken by lust and other deep currents. There is no easy answer, indeed it would be sad if there were, but there is one basic truth to which our attempts at emotional honesty should be directed. Unless you love yourself, you will not be able to love another.

We need others, both in relationships and communities, because honesty is at times hard to bear alone. Here we begin to come full circle; we subscribe to the same values and assumptions, whether right or wrong, because they give us access to each other. People with the same beliefs constitute a community; they have the possibility of understanding each other, of sharing feelings and supporting or potentiating each other.

We cannot always prevent or avoid the things which make us feel bad. Tragedy can strike unexpectedly; losing a loved one can set up an emotional sequence which puts the survivor at risk. Honesty with feelings can reduce this risk by developing a realistic view of ourselves and our role in relation to those events.

All of these elements contribute to confidence, that product of feeling positive about yourself. Without confidence you will not be able to listen and respond to the messages your body is giving you. Nor will you be able to initiate positive action in the depths of your being. As we shall see in the next chapter, your emotional state can exert influence over the responses of your immune system. Feeling positive, and having confidence to act appropriately, can limit the access disease has to your body.

Most of us lack confidence because we grow up subject to the values and assumptions of others. Our conformity to these values will fix our attitudes. As we have already seen, many of the attitudes we acquire are simply wrong, if not positively harmful. Yet there is no denying that the majority of people, in all societies, unquestioningly accept the values and attitudes of their society and are prepared to live by and die for them. In return a range of rewards, real or implied, are offered.

There is a major flaw in the comfort given by passive conformity. As we approach the end of the twentieth century, confronted by an ever-growing number of seemingly insurmountable problems – from the possibility of nuclear annihilation to the increasing incidence of many types of disease – the old wisdom is wearing thin. More and more of us suspect there may be something fundamentally wrong with the assumptions and attitudes we are given.

Breaking free, even to a limited degree, can be difficult. The art is to free yourself from values which act against your best interest, while keeping intact those which help. If we were all the same, it would be possible to write a list, negative on one side, positive on the other. Individual variability invalidates such an approach. For one person an unshakeable belief in a god may be an essential and positive part of life, for another it may be unacceptable and thoroughly depressing. Your job, your home or your children may be essential to your personal fulfilment, or they may be the source of misery and isolation; only you can decide.

You can, of course, produce your own list. If you can write down your life priorities, such as 'improve my immunity to disease', 'feel good about me', 'learn to ski', or whatever, then working on the means to achieve them will inevitably involve some degree of reorientation of values. Your priorities should be totally selfish, they should concern you, not your job, your children, or anyone else – they will benefit later. We are all taught that being selfish is wrong, while in reality it is essential for our integrity as individuals. But selfishness does have another side which we also tend to overlook. We should not try to inflict our self-interested views on others, since they have as much right to their individuality as we have to ours.

Changing values to achieve your own priorities will build confidence. Relying on off-the-shelf answers to off-the-shelf problems caused by off-the-shelf living makes you a victim of those who fill life's shelves. Break that negative cycle, and start to create a positive one by finding yourself. The confidence you will gain is the key to our second objective.

The need to be emotionally honest appears to be in conflict with emotional control. In dealing with other people we have to compromise, and this will sometimes generate conflict within ourselves. This is why it is important to be honest with yourself so that you can decide how honest you want to be with others. Initial honesty gives you the option and a large measure of control.

With total strangers we use manners, and assume that they will do the same, so that we may have social contact with the minimum of exposure of our real feelings. As we get to know people better, we allow more of our real self to be exposed. Within intimate relationships, where trust and the desire for closeness is at its greatest, we expose much more of our inner self.

If you are not sure of yourself you can exert little control over relationships. Being unsure of how you really feel, or repressing an honest expression of your feelings through guilt or upbringing, may allow others to take advantage of you. They may not see it that way, but if someone signals 'yes' (or confusion) when they mean 'no', or vice versa, who is to blame for the resulting misunderstanding?

We find it hard to exert such clear-cut control, seeming to prefer things to take their own course in a mist between our real feelings and unexpressed desires. At times this can lead to situations where we appear either totally out of control or completely dishonest, when we know that neither is really true. It is more likely to be an expression of conflict between ourself, the image our culture gives us of self, and the reflection of ourself gained from others. The tangles of relationships take time to resolve, but resolution is easier if you start with a greater degree of honesty and control.

Total control and total honesty would render us unhuman in a very basic sense. We need an element of capriciousness to maintain stimulation. And our inherent falseness has a positive use. At times life does become almost unbearable; we hear that dull note of mortality struck deep within us. At these times the only option may be to forsake inner reality and flee purposefully to the outer reality of community and culture. Do this in a controlled way. It may help to remember the first rule for learning to ride a bicycle – look at where you want to go, and ignore everything else. Use your knowledge of 'self' and 'non-self' to make choices analogous to those made by your immune system. When appropriate, choose non-self to maintain positive feelings and protect the beauty of your personality. Seek joy and communion outside yourself in the inspiration and energy of others. It is just as real, just as vital, and at times very necessary.

Recharging and building your strength in this way, so that in your turn you may do the same for others, is part of the balance of intellectual and spiritual life that sustains us all. You must be sufficiently in control of yourself to know when you need to draw from the common pool, and when you have something to add to it.

All of the factors we have detailed in this chapter contribute to positive feedback within your being. Good food and physical activity will make you feel good; feeling good will help you sleep; rest will help you become more active, and so on. The aim is to treat yourself as an integrated being, a balanced combination of mind, body and spirit, able to use your capacity to maintain yourself and live the most fulfilling life open to you.

We believe if everyone had a lifestyle which approached the criteria we have described above, then 90 per cent of the population would avoid 90 per cent of the disease which currently afflicts it. Living in this way, with variations to suit individual differences, would create a life dynamic which would make health a life-long norm, rather than the exceptional and transient state experienced today.

As an individual you are unlikely to have to take account of everything we have said. To achieve your instant improvement we would suggest that you assess your current lifestyle, and begin by tackling the area in which you feel you are weakest. This would be the first step, with which all great journeys begin. Work out a plan that will accomplish this, and then add the next step until you have each in balance.

Wherever you start from, you will soon notice a change for the better! In the next chapter we will explain how the right lifestyle directly assists your immune army in its multiplicity of tasks.

Immune Defences

Troops and Training

The body's defence system is very sophisticated. It has an armoury of different weapons and complex control and communication systems to direct and modulate action at every level. It also has a large standing army of specialized fighting troops, the various sorts of white blood cells.

The body of a healthy person contains around a trillion (10,000,000,000,000) white cells, or lymphocytes as they are called. Lymphocytes are carried in the lymph, a colourless liquid that is part of our bloodstream. (*Cyte* = cell, hence lymphocyte = cell of the lymph fluid.) In certain parts of the body, the lymph circulates in a separate system apart from the main bloodstream.

As a fighting machine the immune system has advantages we can only mimic in science fiction stories. It can produce and train billions of new troops as required, create new antibodies to mark enemies, and clone specialized fighters as a rapid response force. Its capacity for information processing is greater than that of our most impressive computers.

While we can describe much of it, our understanding of the immune system is still incomplete. Those aspects which have been most intensively explored are the specialized structures, cells and chemicals which form its more active constituents. In our military analogy, these are the front-line

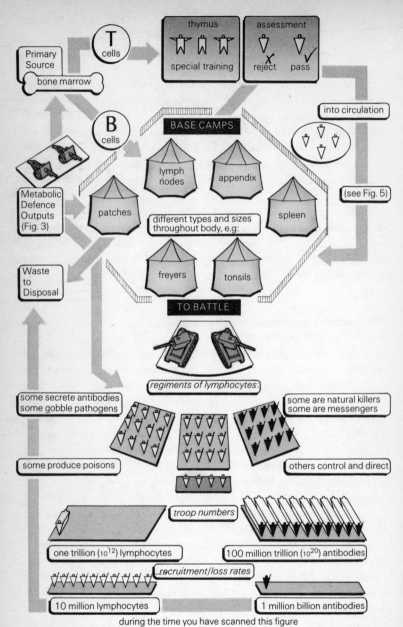

44

Figure 4

troops, the barracks where they develop and mature, the camps where they train and fight, and the weapons they use.

The white-cell troops of the immune army are produced in the bone marrow. From there they move into various camps. Some go to the thymus, an organ that lies just under the breastbone close to the heart, where they undergo the equivalent of officer selection and training. Those that are successful will emerge as T-cells. Meanwhile the rest, mainly B-cells – the privates which make up the bulk of the lymphocyte army – migrate into the circulation and congregate in lymph nodes and other organs of the immune system.

Although lymphocytes are named B- and T-cells, there is no alphabet of immune troops. T-cells are so called because they pass through the thymus. B-cells were named after the *bursa of Fabricius*, an obscure part of avian anatomy where the production of these cells was first observed. The terminology of the immune system is complicated and frequently illogical; but science is often illogical, particularly when it only has a small part of the picture.

Before T-cells are released from the thymus, into the general circulation, they have to pass a strict test. They must demonstrate that they will not attack other healthy cells of the body. To do this they must be able to differentiate between 'self' and 'non-self' molecules in the body. More precisely, they must be sensitive to a range of three-dimensional electron clouds which surround each molecule. The arrangement of the electron cloud projected by a particular molecular form is known as an *antigen* (or sometimes as an *epitope*).

The clumsy term antigen lingers from the time when scientists knew that something was causing the immune system to react at the molecular level by producing *antibodies*, but they were not sure what it was. They described the unknown cause by its effect: *antibody generator* – or antigen for short.

An antigen of a component of the body is a 'self antigen' (perpetuating the clumsiness, since antibodies are not usually produced to the body's own parts). The antigen of a foreign molecule is a 'non-self antigen'. T-cells must make this discrimination reliably. If they get it wrong, the fury of the immune army will be erroneously unleashed on a part of the body it is meant to protect (see pp. 123–4). The vast majority of T-cells fail this crucial test; they are killed by the thymus.

Those successful T-cells in general circulation have a range of tasks. When they pass out from the thymus each is assigned a specific role. Some become Natural Killers, some T-helpers or T-suppressors. In co-operation with each other and specialists from other training camps, they are responsible for front-line operations.

Natural Killers are fine warriors, patrolling the body, seeking out abnormal cells and killing them. They prevent the proliferation of cancer cells and those infected by viruses. They can operate without their victims being marked by antibodies, recognizing the change in form of the membrane of the sick cell. The Natural Killer attaches itself to the cell and appears to deliver a kiss of death, for the cell dies and disintegrates.

T-helpers tell other lymphocytes, including B-cells, to produce antibodies to antigens. T-suppressors, on the other hand, inhibit immune reactions, presumably to keep the battle manageable within its immediate environment.

Among the ranks of the B-cells the tasks are many and varied. Depending on whether instructed by a T-helper or T-suppressor, B-cells can manufacture antibodies to specific antigens. They do this by assembling a string of protein molecules with electron patterns that match those of the antigen. The antibody then attaches to mark the non-self body. The B-cell will divide and subdivide to produce copies of itself to secrete further antibodies to mark other identical antigens. This is essential in the fight against infection, for pathogens tend to multiply at a similar rate. The explosive increase in the number of cells within a lymph node can cause the type of swelling we sometimes notice under our chin during an infection.

Some of these lymphocytes will remember the particular antigen which first stimulated them to produce antibodies. They, and their descendants, will go on producing these antibodies, thus maintaining our immunity to that specific threat. People who were aged over ninety in the 1970s were found to have antibodies to a 'flu from the 1890s circulating in their blood.

Once an antibody is attached to a pathogen, it is marked for destruction. This may happen by the combination being eaten by other white cells, or it may simply be filtered out by the kidneys. Viruses with attached antibodies cannot penetrate cells to reproduce; they are effectively sterilized. The ability to produce large amounts of antibodies in response to the threat of a pathogen is crucial to overwhelming it.

As with all armies there are many variations on the officer/private theme, with specialists evolved to perform variations on the main tasks. The lymphocytes of the immune system are exactly the same; numerous other

46

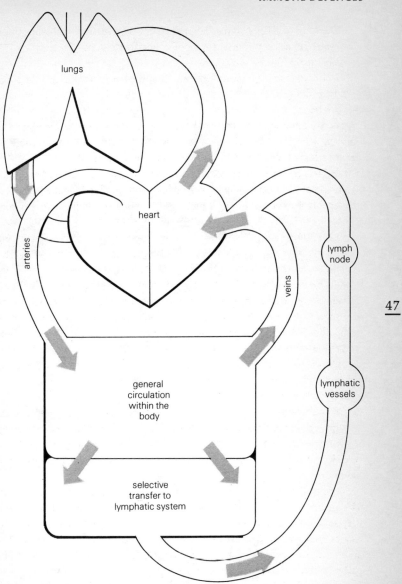

Figure 5

functions carried out by the troops are variations on the theme of marking and destroying enemies.

Barracks and Camps

Various sites around the body are used by the immune system to concentrate its troops. These sites may be concerned with production and training, as with the bone marrow and thymus, or with other parts of the overall protective function.

The names of some camps will be familiar, even if their function is not; the tonsils and adenoids, the spleen and the appendix all contain immune-system tissue. Whereas bone marrow and the thymus have irreplaceable roles in the immune system, some of the other sites do not. This is very fortunate for many people, as surgery has had phases when it was fashionable to remove some of them, often for no better reason than because their function could not be seen, and it was therefore imagined that they did nothing worthwhile. In fact, as a concentration of immune cells, they play a useful role in protecting us.

Lymph nodes are more specialized. They are the small glands, usually about the size of a pea, which swell up in response to an infection. What goes on inside these nodes is not very pleasant (for the enemy); the lymph nodes are part of the lymphatic circulation system. This is a restricted area where only white cells and their prisoners are allowed.

When on patrol in our body, white cells penetrate all our tissues. They can pass from the bloodstream, through the walls of blood vessels when necessary, to get to points where they are needed. Some types of tissue, such as that around joints, are particularly rich in lymphocytes. In this way the activity of the immune system helps preserve one of our basic abilities, that of movement.

The specialized lymphatic circulation system is shown in Figure 5. It has no pump, but is connected with the blood circulation, and draws its power indirectly from the heart. It has an interface with the blood system just under the shoulder blades. Here lymphocytes which have been collected by the special lymphatic vessels are returned to the blood. Looking at this system, one can speculate that in evolutionary terms we may be seeing the development of a separate circulation, one that will eventually have its own heart, or possibly half of the established heart.

48

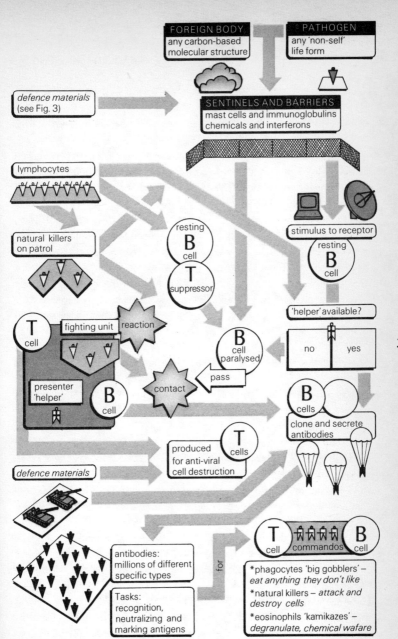

49

Figure 6

As the lymph passes through the lymph nodes it is cleaned by resident white cells. Most of these are B-cells, straight from the bone marrow. They do not need to be very smart, as their job is to gobble up anything they consider to be suspect. The scientific name for this no-nonsense approach is *phagocytosis*, (*phag-* means to eat), so the cells which do this are called phagocytes. The process of gobbling foreign bodies can destroy the gobblers as well, which may be why raw recruits are usually used; 80 millions of them are produced every minute, but they do not survive more than two or three days. The debris from the action in the lymph nodes is returned to the bloodstream to be dealt with by the liver and kidneys.

Figure 6 gives a summary of the deployment of immune-system troops.

Chemical Weapons

White cells can release chemical poisons to kill pathogens. These usually contain highly reactive forms of oxygen, which destroy bacteria by literally burning them away. Other defences involve restricting the access bacteria have to nutrients. Lymphocytes can produce a substance which binds iron, thus making it unavailable to bacteria; without it they cannot reproduce.

When phagocytes (gobblers) are stimulated by an antigen, they may respond by producing *pyrogens*. These cause an increase in temperature, which in turn increases the rate of phagocytosis. Pyrogens can make flesh hot to touch.

There is also an important group of chemicals, made up of proteins, found in lymph and blood serum. These are called *complements*, because of what they do, rather than what they are. There are many types of complement, with many separate functions. They are active in the following processes: coating pathogens to aid the gobblers (a sort of seasoning for the phagocytes); summoning phagocytes to a battle zone; controlling inflammation; making holes in blood vessels to let lymphocytes through; disrupting the membranes of pathogens; contracting muscles; and inducing immune cells to burst and release other chemicals.

Interferons are crucial in preventing each new virus that comes along getting a hold on the body. When we meet a virus for the first time, there is no memory of the appropriate antibody in the immune system. The manufacture and production of sufficient numbers takes time; interferon buys us this time. In warfare it is analogous with the barbed-wired minefield; it tangles up and delays the enemy while the troops get ready to fight.

50

There are various types of interferon, some produced by white cells, and others by body cells which have no specific role in the immune function. One type is produced by cells under attack by viruses. It helps adjacent cells resist viral penetration, and slows down the rate of multiplication of cells where viruses are active. Interferon-treated cells tend to be destroyed by Natural Killers.

The production of interferons causes that characteristic 'under the weather' feeling we get when sickening for something. If the perimeter defences hold and our immune system responds efficiently, that is all we notice. If not, and the infection gets a hold, we will develop the symptoms of the disease.

Because of their value in helping Natural Killers identify targets, some scientists have tried to exploit the properties of interferons. Indeed drug manufacturers have invested many millions in genetically engineered interferon in the hope that it would be another penicillin. So far, trials have proved disappointing in mass-market afflictions, such as the common cold and influenza, although some patients with rare cancers may have been helped.

We believe that the commercial exploitation of interferon could be very dangerous. Every person who is reasonably nourished can produce enough of these substances to fulfil their function. Interferons are sophisticated chemicals in fine balance with the rest of the immune system; this balance has evolved over millennia to meet our needs. It is not the sort of system we should risk upsetting with clumsy intervention, lest in the long run we upset the balance in favour of our enemies. Without barbed wire and mine-fields any enemy could walk right in and prove fatal.

51

Sentinels

On the surfaces of membranes open to the environment, such as those in the nose, intestine and vagina, stand the sentinels whose job is to prevent entry by foes. These are the *mast cells*, and they are similar to immobile B-cells, with capacity for memory and antibody production. Mast cells are also situated at strategic joints and junctions throughout the body.

The special forms of antibody secreted by mast cells are called *immunoglobulins*. Various different types of immunoglobulin are given different letters; while immunoglobulin A (IgA) is particularly plentiful on external membranes, other forms (IgD, IgE, IgG and IgM) are also found. Immuno-globulins are effectively forms of antibody which are specialized to match different types of pathogen; IgA protects mainly against viruses and bacteria, and prevents the entry of potential allergens, while IgE protects us from worms.

Like other types of antibody, the immunoglobulins on mast cells recognize antigens. When a large quantity of antigen which is judged to be dangerous arrives, the mast cells burst, or degranulate, releasing their contents. This poisons pathogens and summons lymphocytes to the area to deal with the threat. Inflammation and soreness are the effects we experience when this happens; the symptoms of allergy result from mistaken degranulation by large numbers of mast cells.

Mast cells contain granules which function as memory chips and record all the substances normally encountered by the sentinel. If allergy or pollu-tion causes many mast cells to degranulate, memory loss can allow the entry of more pollutants or pathogens.

Traitors

Like all armies, the immune system can be a threat to the civil population it is meant to protect. It can make mistakes or run out of control. When this happens, healthy tissue gets damaged. Errors in discrimination can cause body-tissue antigens to be mis-identified as 'non-self'; antibodies are produced against them and they are attacked by the immune army. The result is auto-immune disease. Among the most common results of auto-immune disease are rheumatoid arthritis, ulcerative colitis, juvenile-onset diabetes, and some types of anaemia.

The system of checks and balances created by the interaction of different types of lymphocyte is crucial to reduce the risk of this type of disease. Our immune system will only protect us without causing more than minimal damage if it is capable of precise and reliable discrimination. This is why it is so essential that we do everything possible to avoid overloading or disrupt-ing its memory.

Command and Communication Systems

Overall control over the immune system is the task of the brain. Specialized parts of the brain produce chemical messengers which control the individual cells of the immune system. Lymphocytes have receptors on their surfaces which allow them to receive a variety of chemical messages. Some of these messages come from other immune-system cells, summoning them to battle or stimulating them to action; others are part of the broad coordination of defences by the brain.

Many of these chemical messengers have a range of functions in different parts of the body. Histamine, for example, is involved in inflammation on a local level, in the transmission of nervous impulses within the brain, and in communication between brain and body. Those who have taken anti-histamines for allergy will have experienced the effects of suppressing its multiple functions. Anti-histamines reduce inflammation, and can also cause drowsiness, incoordination and unpredictable emotional changes.

Messages from the brain can intensify or reduce the reactions of any part of the immune system. The command centre is the hypothalamus, which is the part of the brain area that also controls emotional reactions and appetite. It is closely connected both with the cortex, which produces consciousness, thought and our senses, and with the pituitary gland, which controls our hormones. These interconnections allow immunity to be affected by our hormone status, moods and even by our beliefs.

53

If you are angry or afraid, the automatic systems in your brain might anticipate that you could get injured in conflict or a dash to escape from the threat. It would react by gearing up immune defences to maximize resistance to any pathogens to which you might be about to be exposed. To do this, the brain could change the balance of immune activity in favour of T-helpers and against T-suppressors throughout the body. If you are injured, your defences will be strengthened; but in modern society, where the threat is usually symbolic, the result of reducing immune suppression could be an unwelcome flare-up of auto-immune disease or allergy.

The interconnections between mind and body explain why some personality types are more susceptible to immune-system malfunction than others. People who suffer from diseases such as rheumatoid arthritis and ulcerative colitis differ in attitudes and behaviour from their more happy-go-lucky peers and relatives. It seems that the emotional demands they characteristically put on themselves are translated into overreactions by the immune system. Resistance to infection has been found to be related to a wide range of life stress. For example, a study of military cadets showed that those who succumbed to glandular fever were both highly motivated and poor academic achievers; the stress induced by this combination of psycho-logical factors apparently led to reduced immune competence. Similarly, telephone employees who were more dissatisfied with life had more infec-tions. This type of relationship has been found in many studies.

Lonely and unhappy people are particularly prone to infection and other types of illness. Apparently the generals controlling immunity are less in-clined to carry on the struggle for survival when the emotional drive has gone. This effect could result from falling levels of brain neurohormones such as nor-adrenalin and adrenalin. These are important for alertness and a cheerful state of mind. Receptors for these neurohormones have been found on both T- and B-cells, so reactions to infection will be affected by the nor-adrenergic circuits of the brain.

Although there are many complex interactions between different neuro-hormones and our behaviour, some links have clear applications in every-day life. For example, strenuous activity boosts brain levels of nor-adrenalin, inducing a cheerful state of mind and also, presumably, improved antibody production. The type of activity recommended in Chapter 2 will produce benefits on many levels.

54

Another command system is associated with the pineal gland, popularly known as the 'third eye'. The pineal responds to light and darkness, fixing the timing of the rhythms of the body. Secretions from the pineal also modulate immune reactions, so that we respond differently to infections and other immune challenges at different times of the day. The implication of this is that confusing our internal clock – for example, by night work or jet lag – could reduce immunity. Lack of sunlight in winter is known to cause depression; it is also likely that it reduces our resistance to infec-tion.

Resources for Immunity

Motivation

A positive outlook and emotional well-being can have profound benefits for immunity. This is why we consider the last item of the list of lifestyle factors in Chapter 2 to be so important (see pp. 37–41). A lifestyle that matches the timing of the natural rhythms of our bodies will also help the system to work better, improving immunity to infection. Meeting the body's needs for rest, activity and good nutrition will enhance these benefits by helping to maintain emotional stability.

Materials

The physical response to infection described earlier involves the production of millions of new cells. For this, the body needs fuel and the basic building blocks of cells, and the efficient metabolic and delivery systems described earlier.

The immune system requires all the following nutrients: Vitamin A, thiamine, riboflavin, pyridoxine (vitamin B6), vitamin B12, biotin, pantothenic acid, folic acid, vitamin C, vitamin D, vitamin E; zinc, iron, copper, magnesium, selenium. This is why an adequate, balanced diet is so important; taking tablets containing selected vitamins is no substitute for sensible eating.

The most *important* nutrients for high immunity are vitamins A, C and E, and the minerals zinc, iron, magnesium and selenium. The foods recommended in Chapter 2 contain particularly high levels of these nutrients.

Vitamin A is necessary for membrane maintenance and for lymphocyte production and function. Mild vitamin A deficiency impairs the production of immunoglobulins, while severe deficiency causes the thymus and spleen to shrink, producing extreme vulnerability to infection. But this vitamin must be kept in balance because excess depresses immune responses. This is the main reason for getting it from dietary sources, and not expecting benefit from mega-doses.

Vitamin C is crucial because it is used for cell production, especially the creation of new T-cells. It is also used for detoxification and in some chemical weapons. During infection and the early stages of recovery, the body uses vitamin C faster than at other times, so you should endeavour to eat more foods that are rich in this vitamin if you are feeling unwell.

Vitamin E also has many functions in immunity. It is necessary for antibody production and for building new cells, both within the immune system and generally. Along with vitamin C, it plays an important role in clearing the debris produced by the battle against infection.

Zinc is probably the most important mineral in immune function. Because factory farming and food processing reduce the zinc content of foods, zinc deficiency is very common. Zinc is involved in the action of more than seventy enzymes, including those that are crucial to the production of new cells. T-cell numbers fall fast when there is too little zinc in the body, and

55

the thymus suffers. If women are zinc-deficient during pregnancy, their offspring can suffer permanently impaired immune function. Vegetarians who adopt a normal diet minus the meat, rather than eating organic whole-foods, are especially likely to go short of zinc. Fortunately it is very easy both to detect and to treat the problem using a zinc sulphate solution, sold as 'Zincatest'. To those who have no need of zinc, the solution tastes horrible, while those who need zinc may not be able to taste it at all.

Iron is crucial to the production of enzymes used to destroy bacteria. In addition, many enzymes necessary for normal cell metabolism and detoxifica-tion contain iron. The iron-binding proteins that act to deprive bacteria of this important mineral paradoxically contain iron themselves; and red blood cells depend on iron for the 'haem' part of the haemoglobin that delivers oxygen to the whole of the body. Iron deficiency seems relatively less common than deficiencies of other important minerals, except among the seriously undernourished and vegetarians who fail to eat enough dark green vegetables. Iron excess is as likely to be a problem in Britain, at least among meat-eaters; like excesses of most minerals, this depresses immune function.

Magnesium is often deficient in British soils and in modern foods, and surveys have shown that few people get enough dietary magnesium. Mag-nesium forms an essential part of complement and is necessary for the production of lymphocytes. It is also essential to the cardio-vascular system, protecting against spasm in the blood vessels.

Selenium deficiency is particularly dangerous when vitamin E intake is also inadequate. These two nutrients act together in detoxification and the removal of reactive oxygen-containing compounds. If this process does not operate at sufficient speed, T-cells can be coated with inhibitors derived from these reactive compounds, and thus rendered ineffective.

Finally, the cells and chemicals which must be manufactured at such a tremendous rate to meet any potential threat are made up of *proteins*. A diet that contains too little protein will undermine immunity. Relative protein deficiency, with protein loss from the body, is common with many low-calorie diets. Starving or malnourished people are always highly vulnerable to infection, partly because of a lack of available protein. There is no need, however, for people eating a mixed diet that supplies sufficient total quan-tities of food (see Chapter 2) to be specifically concerned about protein, for it occurs in a great many types of food including the staples that are common to both mixed and vegetarian diets.

Clearing the Debris

The aspect of warfare that armies and commanders tend not to consider is the chaos produced on the battlefield. In the body, tidying up this mess is as crucial as being able to win the battle, for damaged tissue will not be capable of functioning satisfactorily until everything has returned more or less to normal. It is not unusual for the destruction caused by immune reactions to be greater than that due to the pathogens which precipitated the battle. Indeed, in allergic and auto-immune reactions, there may be no pathogens at all, merely mis-identified stimuli that would have done no damage if the system had ignored them.

Whatever the origin of the conflict, it is always necessary to remove debris, to make safe the poisons produced by the protagonists, and to rebuild the tissue in the area.

While surviving lymphocytes may leave the battle zone, great quantities of dead cells are sometimes expelled from the body through channels created for them. We experience such activities as spots or boils which rise through the skin to burst open and spill their contents into the oxygen-rich atmosphere which should kill any remaining pathogens. The same strategy is used by the immune system to rid the body of large foreign bodies such as deep splinters and bits of metal that accidentally get embedded in our tissues.

Chemical debris is broken down by enzyme systems which operate throughout the body, but which are concentrated in the liver. Detoxification systems within the liver deal with all types of debris, whatever its source. The same systems break down the by-products of infection as well as chemicals that arrive in our blood from the air, from food, drink, or drugs; they take apart unwanted hormones, worn-out cells, and everything else that needs to be disposed of in the most efficient way possible.

Although these systems are highly sophisticated and capable of dealing with a high loading, their capacity is limited. Most of us have experienced the misery of a hangover, the product of a liver overloaded with alcohol. If the body is expected to deal with debris from infection at the same time as a heavy load of chemicals, drugs, or alcohol, this point of overload will be more quickly reached. There will inevitably be inefficiency and delay in the cleaning-up process. In extreme circumstances, the liver can be damaged by the poisons it is unable to detoxify with sufficient speed. If it is having to deal with attack by a virulent organism at the same time, long-term damage may result.

The products that result from the detoxification process are often large molecules or *antibody–antigen complexes*. These are attached to special substances which act like biological wheelbarrows to move unwanted material through the bloodstream to the kidneys. Here the wheelbarrows tip their contents into the urine for disposal. The kidneys are at risk when this happens too fast because the concentration of toxins or large antibody–antigen complexes can rise too high. The system of delicate tubules where the blood is filtered can be overwhelmed. The kidneys of elderly people are particularly likely to be damaged by medicinal drugs if they, or their metabolic by-products, arrive in high concentrations; while antibody–antigen complexes produced by immune reactions are most likely to cause kidney failure in young people. When drugs are given for infection, the kidneys suffer double jeopardy. The risk of kidney failure in these circumstances seems to be particularly high with antibiotics of the tetracyclin group and the sulphonamides.

Kidney function can be assisted by drinking plenty of *pure* water. This reduces the concentration of potentially dangerous substances. Dehydration is a particular risk when high temperature (whether the product of fever, prolonged activity, or a hot environment) or diarrhoea causes increased elimination of water from the body. Drink as much water as possible under such circumstances, so that the urine always remains pale in colour.

Recovery from damage involves reconstruction and repair, which is essential to protect the area from renewed onslaught by pathogens. These require much the same support systems as the immune response did, for the logistics of the situation are basically the same. What is necessary are new cells, built primarily of proteins and micronutrients, using oxygen and carbohydrate for construction energy.

For rapid healing, body and mind need to be at rest. Rest provides a hormonal environment which is favourable to repair. Good nutrition, with attention to the nutrients listed above, especially zinc and vitamin A, provides the materials. Poor healing is often a sign of poor diet, although it can also result from inadequate blood supply due to smoking or long-term inactivity.

Provided the basic needs are met, all that is then required is time – more as we get older, for the rebuilding process slows down as the years accumulate.

Mercenaries

Vaccination

The process of vaccination is intended to provoke the immune system to produce antibodies to a specific infection. The vaccine contains antigens which are also characteristic of the pathogen. Because they are derived from dead or denatured pathogens, vaccination does not cause the disease, but merely an appropriate immune response. The immune system will usually retain the memory of antigens in the vaccine for some years, perhaps a lifetime. A vaccinated individual has a better chance of resisting a pathogen carrying the same antigens because the memory gives lymphocytes a head start.

Vaccination has proved very valuable in the fight against some diseases. The greatest triumph of the method has been in the total suppression of smallpox by a world-wide campaign orchestrated by the World Health Organization. Smallpox vaccination teams travelled into the most remote areas of the world to ensure that the disease would not spread from any neglected centre.

It was the desire to achieve protection from smallpox that led to the adoption of vaccination hundreds of years before the virus that caused it was isolated. It was known that smallpox would strike an individual only once. But, according to country lore, milkmaids who had suffered from cowpox were safe from smallpox. Milkmaids were known for their perfect complexions, free from pits and hollows left by the disfiguring pox. But their hands were another matter; there the signs of the cowpox, a mild disease, were to be found. Somehow this seemed to protect them from smallpox.

Edward Jenner became famous for his experiments with the use of inoculate from the cowpox sore to vaccinate other people. They developed a mild attack of the cowpox, but did not suffer smallpox. After trials on orphans and convicts, the method was used to protect the gentry, and eventually millions of others. Cowpox and smallpox viruses are sufficiently similar to share many antigens, so immunity to one provides immunity to the other. This is a rare situation. It happens more often that viruses producing the same disease do *not* share antigens that permit cross-immunity. Some viruses change their antigenic nature – the shape of their coat – at frequent intervals, and so evade the antibodies. This is one of the limitations of vaccination.

Stimulating the immune system artificially in this way does have hazards, and benefits have to be weighed against risks before mass vaccination programmes are carried out. Sometimes risks are ignored or unrecognized, as in Africa where children are vaccinated using needles which carry the AIDS virus. Even without such hazards, vaccination will not work on people who are not sufficiently well nourished for their bodies to mount an adequate immune response. It could merely help to weaken them further.

Antibiotics

Antibiotics are seen by many as medicine's greatest triumph. They are the archetypal 'magic bullets' which kill the pathogens without harming the host. Many people imagine that some variant on the antibiotic theme will be discovered to provide a cure for every infectious condition. Regrettably, these dreams are built on a distorted picture of antibiotics. They are, in our military analogy, unreliable mercenaries, no substitute for an effective immune system.

Antibiotics are medicines used to kill living organisms. The difference between modern antibiotics and the sort of poisons that doctors used to prescribe a hundred years ago is that ours are more selective in their poisoning propensities. They have some degree of preference for bacteria, or worms or whatever, rather than our own body cells. Penicillin, the most selective anti-bacterial drug yet developed, is also the safest; yet around twenty people die each year in Britain from anaphylactic shock due to penicillin.

Anti-viral drugs, although offering some relief from some viral infections, are of little use against viruses inside cells. Virus infections cannot be cured by outside agents; we rely on our immune systems.

Disruptors

Most of the substances that disrupt our immune defences enter our bodies while we fulfil the fundamental requirements for continuing life. Air, food, drink and other people are the vectors of disease and form the disruptors of our defences which aid it. Other important sources of immune disruption are medical treatment and radiation.

Air Pollution

Air pollution is particularly damaging. Our lungs are not equipped to cope with the sort of pollution generated by our industrial way of life. In the primeval forests and grasslands where our ancestors evolved, there was very little that could pollute the air; volcanic eruptions and forest fires would have been too rare to stimulate the development of specific protective systems. The mechanisms that protect us from dust particles (hair-lined nostrils, mucus, and the sneeze reflex) are not able to cope with the pollutants that predominate today.

Tobacco smoke

We have already described cigarette smoke as the pollutant that causes more damage than any other. Its hazards are of many kinds, operating at many levels to produce an extensive and grim picture.

At the respiratory membranes, tobacco smoke stimulates the over-production of mucus in a vain attempt to wash the tars and poisons away. The effectiveness of this defence measure is limited because the smoke paralyses the cilia, tiny hairs which should keep this mucus on the move, washing pathogens away from the cells. We cough to remove excess mucus, but cigarette smoke disrupts the cough reflex. The result is that this mucus acts like unchanged bandages, trapping pathogens and toxins on the surface of the respiratory membranes.

Cigarette smoke contains hundreds of different chemical compounds. In addition to the products of burning tobacco, there are chemicals used in cigarette manufacture and tobacco treatment. Each of these will be identified by the mast cells which line the respiratory tract and they will stimulate antibody production. The more the immune-system cells have to devote themselves to coping with cigarette smoke, the less capacity they have available to prevent entry by pathogens.

Neither mucus nor antibodies can prevent poisons in the smoke from reaching the surface of the cells lining the respiratory passages. It is here that they begin to exert their poisonous effects. Not only do the chemicals in tobacco smoke irritate and inflame, but they can penetrate inside living cells and damage the genetic material that controls them. This is what sets off the growth of cancers in the respiratory tract that are characteristic of smokers.

The depth to which the carcinogenic chemicals in cigarette smoke penetrate depends on the depth of inhalation. People who habitually inhale deeply tend to develop lung cancers, while those who hardly inhale at all are more likely to develop throat and bronchial cancers. Predictably, those who chew tobacco develop mouth and gullet cancers, while those who snort tobacco snuff develop cancers of the nose and sinuses.

Non-smokers who have the misfortune to be exposed to smokers are also at risk. Non-smoking spouses of smokers run about double the risk of cancer, compared with non-smoking couples. Family members of smokers, particularly children, have higher rates of infection.

Some components of tobacco smoke are carried through the respiratory membranes into the bloodstream. They end up in the liver, where they can affect the balance of the two stages of detoxification carried out by liver enzymes. The activity of the first group of enzymes involved in detoxification can be so greatly enhanced that the second stage cannot keep pace. The result is increased production of 'reactive intermediates' – substances which are actually more toxic than those with which the body started. This means that cigarette smoke is capable of making other dangerous substances into much greater threats than would otherwise be the case. Liver detoxifying capacity is thus reduced both directly and indirectly by the action of cigarette smoke.

One of the many poisons in cigarette smoke is carbon monoxide. This enters the bloodstream without hindrance, and its effect is to block the oxygen-carrying capacity of the red blood cells. This disrupts metabolism throughout the body, reducing the effectiveness of the immune system which depends on oxygen for many aspects of its function.

The hazard of carbon monoxide is enhanced by the action of nicotine on the nervous system. Nicotine shuts down the circulation in the limbs and skin by reducing the carrying capacity of blood vessels. This means that delivery of nutrients to the extremities is chronically impeded in regular smokers, so defences against damage and infection are reduced. Chronic ulcers and gangrene can be the results.

One poison in cigarette smoke which has particular relevance to the immune system is cadmium. It acts as a zinc antagonist, disrupting the immune system at every point where zinc is involved, notably in tissue-building and production of lymphocytes.

Vehicle Emissions

Exhaust gases from motor vehicles have replaced coal smoke as the primary source of air pollution in most cities. Like cigarette smoke, these gases cause damage at every level of the immune system. All societies share a blind spot for this health disruptor; people everywhere love their tin and chrome extensions. But we pay a high price in health for our fantasies.

Car exhausts contain oxides of nitrogen, carbon monoxide and lead compounds. Diesel vehicle exhausts contain sulphur compounds (including sulphuric acid), and carbon particles. Both petrol and diesel engines produce a variety of hydrocarbons, especially when they are not running as efficiently as they should. Some of these compounds – in particular, benzo-(a)-pyrene – are known to be carcinogenic.

At the respiratory membranes, the damage caused by the hydrocarbons produced by motor vehicles is similar to that caused by the tars from cigarettes. They impair the function of the mast cells and increase the risk of cancers in the respiratory system. City dwellers are more at risk of respiratory cancers than people living in the country; for people who both live in the city and smoke cigarettes, the risks are multiplied. Vehicle exhaust is the major source of excess hazard in cities and we can anticipate a growing number of cancer deaths, despite the decreasing popularity of cigarettes, as our use of motor vehicles continues to rise.

Bladder cancer is a common effect of absorption of dangerous synthetic chemicals which has also been linked with diesel fumes. Drivers of diesel vehicles in London have an unusually high incidence of this cancer.

The effects of exhaust fumes have been studied less than those of cigarettes. Nevertheless, the similarity in the type of hazard suggests that resistance to all types of respiratory infection would be reduced in people exposed to vehicle exhausts. Lowered resistance compounds the effects of close contact with a large number of other people, among whom virus infections will readily spread. Respiratory allergies, such as hay fever, have been shown to be more common among people living in towns; these are also predictable reactions to membrane damage and mast cell overload.

The parallels between vehicle exhausts and cigarettes go further. Both also produce carbon monoxide. It has been estimated that an hour's exposure to prime London traffic does the same amount of damage to the body's oxygen-carrying capacity as smoking four cigarettes. Whereas cigarette smoke contains cadium, car exhaust fumes deliver lead, also a zinc antagonist. Lead accumulates in our bodies, damaging the brain and blood, and impairing immunity. Although we can get lead from many sources, air pollution is the most dangerous; relatively little of the lead in our food is taken into the body, but virtually all of the lead in the air we breathe will enter the bloodstream.

Lead is capable of mimicking zinc, iron, calcium, magnesium, and copper in the body. Thus it can disable the enzymes that control virtually all aspects of our metabolism. In view of this, it is not surprising that lead poisoning has been linked with premature death from a very wide range of causes. People of all ages are damaged by lead, but children are most at risk: they suffer progressive brain damage as lead accumulates in the nervous system. There is no safe level of lead intake. The EEC has acknowledged the hazard but car manufacturers will be allowed to continue producing vehicles that require leaded petrol until 1991; it is obvious that lead will continue to be added to petrol for some decades yet. The slowness of government action on this issue is a grim reflection of the real priorities of our politicians.

Resistance to the ill-effects of lead can be improved somewhat by good nutrition. High intakes of micronutrients, especially zinc, will tend to prevent substitution by lead in the tissues; while apples and pears help prevent absorption. A good diet – as described in Chapter 2 – is especially important for city dwellers.

Avoiding exhaust fumes entirely is impossible, but we can reduce our exposure to them by choosing to walk, run or cycle along quiet routes and paths and by avoiding the use of motor vehicles whenever possible. We should never ignore the health costs of apparently convenient mobility.

Air Pollution by Industry

Industrial air pollution is known to cause many cancers. These occur both among people who work in certain industries and among those who have the misfortune to live close to polluting factories. The range of hazards is wide, but the greatest danger seems to be associated with the petro-chemical industry. Recent surveys of American counties where there are large chemical installations have revealed excessive mortality among men from cancer, particularly of the bladder, lung and liver.

As with most carcinogens, the effects of these chemicals will multiply the risks posed by other environmental hazards. For example, exposure to airborne asbestos fibres produces a lung cancer rate among smokers that is more than ninety times higher than that among non-smokers.

Little is known about the carcinogenic effects of most synthetic chemicals and the by-products of their production. It usually takes at least two or three decades to discover that a particular substance causes cancer. By this time, many people will have been irreversibly damaged by it. Yet more and more substances are being released into the general environment without any serious attempt to monitor their effects. All add to the load on our immune defences; all make us more susceptible to many forms of immune breakdown.

Agribusiness, the industry that has largely replaced what we once knew as farming, regularly and repeatedly pollutes the air with poisons. Some of these are known to damage the immune system. One in particular, aldicarb,

65

has been the cause of recent concern in the United States, where researchers at the University of Wisconsin have discovered direct damage to lymphocytes which produces effects similar to AIDS. Yet at the same time as experts and environmentalists call for the withdrawal of aldicarb, the leading brand of this pesticide is intensively advertised on television.

Crop spraying and fumigation produces allergic reactions in many people who live near chemical-dependent farming businesses. Asthma is one of many well-documented effects of pesticide drifting into homes and gardens. Toxicity testing of pesticides leaves much to be desired. There is a general lack of long-term assessment, and the actual effects on human populations are usually unknown. It is known that many pesticides interact with one another and with other substances in the body; the result is likely to be synergistic (multiplicative) effects of potential carcinogens and immune-system poisons. This is the pattern that characterizes such compounds as have been studied. Yet there are no warnings, and apparently no concern, about the use of many different chemicals in close succession.

Many pesticides have been linked with increased incidence of cancers in animal experiments. Examples include dichlorvos, used in homes and gardens as well as in agriculture and food storage; 2,4,5-T, a herbicide used in large quantities by the Forestry Commission; captan, a popular fungicide; and dieldrin, a particularly hazardous insecticide which has been banned in many countries but, like many other risky chemicals, is still used in Britain.

Incineration

Recognition of the hazards of coal smoke led to the introduction of the Clean Air Acts, which have reduced the mortality from bronchitis and related diseases in British cities. Today, the trend is towards incineration of a lower volume of substances which are potentially more dangerous to the immune system. We desperately need a new Clean Air Act.

Burning plastic produces foul-smelling and dangerous fumes. Yet many individuals and small companies casually burn plastics and there is very little that can be done to stop them. The only legal requirement is that *black* smoke should not be produced; but many waste-disposal companies get around this outmoded restriction by burning at night, when the colour of the smoke is less obvious and the environmental health officer has gone home.

Incinerators which process household rubbish should reach a sufficiently high temperature to break down dangerous substances such as polycyclic hydrocarbons to their basic constituents. If this is done, harmless gases such as carbon dioxide and water vapour can be produced. But if the air intake is inadequate, or the temperature too low, or the operators careless, then the products of combustion are likely to include dangerous dioxins, chemicals of the same type as those which caused disease and widespread environmental poisoning when a chemical plant exploded at Seveso.

Waste products from the pharmaceutical industry form a cocktail of dangerous chemicals. Too hazardous for disposal by normally accepted methods, these are burnt at sea on special boats, producing air pollution that will spread with the wind. The advantage of such an operation to the pollutors is that the effects of their actions will be less readily traced to their source than when such fumes are generated in areas where people may protest.

Even after death, we continue to pollute our environment. The coffins in which cemeteries burn bodies are no longer made of wood, which produces few toxic by-products; today, the reconstituted wood is bound together with plastics. The coffin's linings and coatings are also of synthetic materials which give off toxic fumes when burnt at the temperatures at which most cemetery furnaces operate.

67

Household Pollution

In homes that are closely sealed against heat loss, the smells that are generated indoors become more concentrated. Fresh air is an expensive commodity; most people today seem to prefer synthetic substitutes delivered from sprays. Deodorants and room perfumes come in a range of synthetic forms, delivering air pollution on a domestic scale to further confuse our immune defences.

The most hazardous of the domestic air pollutants are the pesticides. Fly killers in the home can induce allergic and toxic reactions; some contain chemicals such as dichlorvos which are known to cause cancer in animals. They should be avoided completely.

Food Pollution

The pollution of food comes primarily from the manufacturers' desire to 'add value' – i.e. profit – to their products. Adding value means substituting chemicals for nutrients. This can harm the immune system because the mast cells which line the gut walls have to identify and respond appropriately to every one of the chemicals which enter our bodies in food. These cells control the input of nutrients, selectively absorbing those that we require while rejecting others. If the system works efficiently, it can both protect us from poisons and ensure that our need for minerals is met if at all possible. But as with other delicately balanced systems, overloading is liable to disrupt its smooth operation.

Even when chemicals arrive in our bodies in minute quantities, the cells of the immune system will respond to them; and the potential for overload of immune memory and consequent mis-identification is increased. It is entirely predictable that the increased consumption of processed and polluted food would lead to a massive upsurge of food allergy and food-related illness. The number of different chemicals in the average processed diet is unknown. There are no controls over many of them. Only the manufacturers know what 'flavourings' go into their products; or what residues of process chemicals may be left behind. Manufacturers are probably too busy to concern themselves with the effects of these substances on the immune system.

Even if we set out to avoid named additives (such as those with E numbers, listed on some labels), we cannot know about those whose names do not appear. The consumer is not likely to be aware that frozen cauliflower pieces may have been steeped in whitening chemicals before packaging, or that the wheat used in bakery products may have been fumigated with the liver poison, carbon tetrachloride. Yet the immune system will detect the residues of these substances and will have to react to them.

Pesticide and drug residues in food are widespread and difficult to detect. Those whose sense of taste has not been deadened by zinc deficiency may know the revolting flavour of pesticide residues on fruit. At least one third of the fruit and vegetable samples tested in a study by the Association of Public Analysts were found to have detectable pesticide residues; 10 per cent of fruit and 20 per cent of vegetables on sale in Britain were over the Ministry of Agriculture's Reporting Limits.

The only way to avoid pesticide residues is to eat organic. All other produce must be assumed to have been sprayed at least a dozen times.

Direct damage to the immune system is not a recognized effect of any food additive. However, some are known to trigger allergic reactions in up to 10 per cent of the population. Asthma, eczema and hyperactivity are particularly common effects of synthetic food colours (especially those falling between E102 and E133) and the benzoate preservatives (E212 to E219). A full list of additives known to be linked with these problems is given in Maurice Hanssen's *E for Additives*.

A substance that is not generally recognized as a food additive is processed (white) sugar. Refined sugar is a chemical compound which can disrupt immune function through the induction of abnormal increases in blood-sugar levels. This impairs lymphocyte, and particularly phagocyte, function, reducing resistance to infection. Low blood-sugar levels (hypoglycaemia) are also associated with reduced immune competence. The most common reason for both of these conditions is the consumption of sugar. Years of habitual sugar consumption causes diabetes in susceptible people. Diabetes is defined by an excess of sugar in the blood, and is frequently detected in elderly people when doctors look for underlying reasons for repeated infection and healing difficulties. In these cases, the sugar-induced metabolic problem is revealed by poor immune function.

A potentially dangerous pollutant to which we may be exposed when we chew is mercury. This toxic metal is not a common direct pollutant in food, except when people eat seed grain coated with mercury pesticides or seafood from estuaries polluted with industrial wastes. For most of us, its main source is the amalgam in our teeth.

Mercury can reduce the number of lymphocytes available for immunity. Like cadmium and lead, it can act as a zinc antagonist, preventing enzymes from doing their normal work. Individuals differ in sensitivity to mercury and it is difficult to assess the potential hazard of amalgam fillings; for most people, replacement of all amalgam fillings may not be justified. Women should not undergo any dental treatment involving amalgam when they are pregnant, for the increase in body mercury that occurs with dental work could damage the baby's developing immune system. This is still a disputed area and the evidence of damage to immunity due to amalgam fillings is not yet strong; research continues but it is impeded by opposition from vested interests. However, the use of a toxic metal in teeth is inherently hazardous and in our view should be discontinued now that safer substitutes are available.

Drink

Although water is essential to health, British tap water is more likely to disrupt immune defences. The damage begins, ironically, with chlorine treatment designed to protect us from infection. Chlorine is a highly reactive element which damages cell membranes directly and readily forms compounds which can further damage the digestive tract. Just as chlorine kills microscopic life in water, so it can disrupt the microscopic life-forms in our gut, reducing the availability of their valuable output.

Carcinogenic chlorine compounds such as chloroform have been found in drinking water. These pollutants will tend to increase the risk of allergic reactions, although they occur in quantities too small to pose more than the slightest theoretical risk of cancer.

Organic compounds in water supplies take many forms. In London, the average cup of tea passes through seven people between source and sea. This process leads to the addition of drug and hormone metabolites in the water, along with all the many complex substances that go down our drains. Filters and other treatment systems will remove some but not all of these substances. The concentration may be small, but the body will respond nevertheless.

Water in many country areas is not likely to be much more pleasant. It is susceptible to pollution by run-off from agribusiness fields. Recent concern has focussed on nitrates because of the sheer quantity that can get into the water supply and the known harm they can cause. In intensively farmed parts of Britain, the nitrate levels in water break EEC requirements. The government has responded by sanctioning the breach of European law, because measures to protect the public are considered too expensive. Run-off from fields will also contain pesticides and other chemicals used in agriculture. While the quantities of these substances in our drinking water may not be high, we should not assume them to be harmless.

Alcoholic drinks are generally known to be potentially hazardous, at least in quantity. Today the main problem for many people is not the alcohol itself, but the other rubbish that is added to it. Preservatives in wine (usually sulphites) are common causes of allergy and will produce very nasty hangovers in sensitive people. Some brewers have added chemicals to their beers to produce hangovers, to persuade naive drinkers of the potency of their products. The hangover is a straightforward symptom of poisoning. The liver gets overloaded with toxic substances in the drink and the nausea, headaches, and general misery that result are signs of this overload. Clearly, when the body's detoxification systems are preoccupied in this way, we are rendered more vulnerable to any other sources of damage.

Alcohol, although linked with a range of cancers, is probably not in itself carcinogenic. It does cause liver damage which may progress to cancer, but it may contribute to disease in other ways. Alcohol can help other carcinogens to penetrate deep into cells, interacting, for example, with cigarette smoke to increase the risk of mouth and oesophageal cancers.

Radiation

Radiation disrupts the immune system primarily by damaging the chromosomes on which each cell's genetic information is recorded. The body is most vulnerable to hazards of this kind when cell division is fastest and the errors in genetic information get multiplied before they can be corrected. The blood cells on which the immune system depends are the fastest-multiplying cells in the body; so it is entirely predictable that radiation would be particularly dangerous to immunity.

When radiation affects the whole body, as it does when people are exposed to leaks from the nuclear industry, it can produce leukaemia. This is a cancer-like disease of the bone marrow, where white cells proliferate uncontrollably but fail to mature. One result is that the individual becomes prone to all forms of infection; another is that red blood cells fail to be produced in adequate numbers, causing extreme weakness and problems with blood clotting.

The incidence of leukaemia has been rising steadily during the course of this century. It tripled between 1930 and 1955, when X-rays were much used; at the time it was not recognized that X-rays could cause leukaemia. Today, while we have become more circumspect about the use of X-rays, the leukaemia incidence associated with the nuclear industry and our nuclear weapons programme is disturbingly high. A twenty-one-year government survey of the areas around fourteen nuclear installations (the publication of which has been long delayed) reported in the *Guardian*, 17 February 1987, reveals that the protesters' claims are justified; there are significant excesses of deaths from leukaemia in such locations. Earlier surveys have uncovered excess rates of other types of cancer, especially in people employed in the nuclear industry or exposed to the effects of nuclear weapons.

Radiation, like most things affecting our health, is a political question. The disaster at Chernobyl changed many people's perception of the reality of nuclear power in a way which Sellafield, with its slow tide of pollution in the sea spreading for thousands of square miles round the source in Cumbria,

71

would not have done. The results of both, one an accident, the other intentional, are the same: a predictable increase in cancer and immune disruption for generations to come.

The X-ray story is one of the less well-known disasters of modern medicine. When doctors want to shrink a part of the body without cutting it, or to sterilize some part of the body, they can use high doses of X-rays. This method is still employed in cancer treatment, despite the immune depression that it induces. It used to be used in a range of medical procedures that are now known to be not only irrational but extremely harmful.

From the 1930s, X-rays were given to the ovaries of women with benign menopausal bleeding. In one study of the effects of this treatment, 2,000 such women were identified from Scottish radiotherapy centres. By the early 1970s, a quarter had died; leukaemia deaths were two and a half times the expected rate. Other cancers of pelvic sites were also increased. An even more dramatically elevated death-rate was found among people given radiotherapy for the spinal disease, ankylosing spondylitis. They had eleven times the usual rate of deaths from leukaemia and the blood disease aplastic anaemia, and twice the usual death-rate from other cancers. In addition, they had more deaths than expected from a wide variety of other conditions, including infections; though the authors of the report considered that these might be associated with suffering from ankylosing spondylitis, rather than the treatment given for it.

In the United States, X-ray treatment achieved an even greater level of popularity. When World War II ended, the US electronics industry found itself with excess capacity so it turned to the production of small X-ray machines. Within a few years virtually every doctor's office had one, and a great number of minor complaints were treated with X-rays.

One of the more regrettable uses of X-rays was to shrink the thymus gland in infants. During the first year of life, before immunity has fully developed, babies can suffer many colds; coincidentally, the thymus is relatively large. Doctors, blaming the large thymus for colds just as they blamed large tonsils for sore throats, would casually damage these infants' immune systems. In 1950, when, according to paediatrician Ronald Glaser, 'therapeutic low-dose radiation had become almost a routine part of paediatric care', an association between irradiation of the thymus and thyroid cancer was reported. Nevertheless, the method continued to be used. Over the next decade, the incidence of thyroid cancer doubled. We have no doubt that this represents just one aspect of the widespread damage that must have been done by such treatment.

Drugs

Disruption of the immune system by medicine is commonplace. Usually, the damage is relatively minor and temporary. When it is severe, the justification given is that the disease would have been even worse than the effects of treatment. Naturally, this is a matter of judgement, though few patients dare question medical opinion.

Deliberate suppression of immune reactions is essential to the success of transplant surgery. Unless recipients of transplants take drugs to prevent their bodies rejecting their new organs, their immune systems would quickly destroy them. Even with immunosuppression, rejection does occur quite frequently; the importance of tissue matching is to reduce the risk of rejection to a treatable level.

The effects of immunosuppression are entirely predictable. Transplant recipients cannot expect to live normal, healthy lives even if the transplanted organ works perfectly. They are especially vulnerable to infections and cancers; in fact, the types of diseases that are now seen in AIDS patients were frequently observed among transplant recipients. The cancers they suffer are often of the immune system, for example B-cell lymphomas. Transplant patients used to be almost the only people to develop the now familiar Kaposi's sarcoma. They have a twenty- to forty-fold increase in liver cancers and an almost fifty-fold increase in non-Hodgkin's lymphoma. They are also more likely to suffer cervical cancers. The excess risk of cancer becomes apparent within six months of the transplant; the more intense the immunosuppression used, the greater the risk of cancer.

All these types of cancer are thought to have links with virus infections. It seems that viruses could cause many human cancers; the only reason they do not do so under normal circumstances is that our immune defences (in particular, our Natural Killer cells) protect us. We disrupt these defences at our peril. Those people who suggest that immunosuppression is an appropriate way of dealing with auto-immune diseases such as juvenile-onset diabetes cannot have given serious consideration to the consequences.

Immunosuppression is generally considered justified when serious disease is being treated. It is a frequent effect of most types of anti-cancer therapy. Predictably cytotoxic drugs, intended to kill rapidly-dividing cancer cells, also damage the cells of the bone marrow and thus disrupt immunity. Leukaemias now develop as side-effects of treatment for cancer.

Many drugs cause less severe forms of immunosuppression. Of the commonly used medicines, steroid preparations are probably the worst in this respect. Predominantly used for their anti-inflammatory and anti-allergic effects, they are intended to reduce immune reactions. Naturally, they also increase the risk of infection.

Ironically, antibiotics seem capable of causing some degree of immune suppression. The most dangerous is chloramphenicol, a drug rarely used in Britain because it can damage the bone marrow, causing a fatal blood disease called aplastic anaemia. Other drugs which can induce anaemia through immune reactions include quinine, penicillins, cephalosporins, and methyldopa.

Oral contraceptives have many effects which can disrupt immunity both directly and indirectly. Pill users are more likely to suffer from infections, allergies and cancers. The damage to the immune system is likely to be more severe the longer a woman takes the Pill, and it can persist for many years after use has ended. But each woman's response to the Pill is individual, and its effects on the immune system are complex, one aspect sometimes balancing another; so while it causes serious damage to some women, others suffer no ill-effects.

Pill-related infection problems are particularly marked in the sex organs, since they are most responsive to hormone changes. Sores on the cervix (cervical erosions) due to the Pill allow easier access for viruses, including those that can cause cervical cancer. The current genital herpes epidemic may be largely due to the Pill; surveys of Pill users by the Royal College of General Practitioners show that resistance to viral infection generally is depressed. Fungus (candida, or thrush) infection of the vagina is also common because the Pill disrupts the normal membrane defences.

Cancers which have been linked with Pill use include those of the cervix, ovaries, breast, endometrium, urinary tract, skin and liver. Women who both smoke and take the Pill are more likely to develop lung cancer. It appears that the Pill interacts with other, more potent carcinogens, producing the now-familiar synergism, or multiplicative effect.

Allergic reactions, including rhinitis, hay fever, food allergy and chemical sensitivity, are more common among Pill users and ex-Pill users; also some auto-immune diseases such as ulcerative colitis. However, rheumatoid arthritis can sometimes be relieved by hormones in the Pill.

The Pill produces many metabolic changes including alterations in liver enzyme activity which increase toxicity problems caused by other drugs, and presumably environmental toxins too. This problem is exacerbated by zinc depletion, which frequently develops when women take the Pill.

Other People

Both isolation and overcrowding can alter immune reactions. But even in animal studies, the effects vary with the species, the particular pathogen and the precise conditions of the experiment. In the context of complex human societies, it is much more difficult to define the precise parameters that are important.

Simple interaction with many other people obviously increases the risk of infectious disease. Other people are the breeding grounds for human pathogens, and the more people there are, the better the conditions for producing greater numbers of pathogens. However, this straightforward hazard is compounded by other more subtle forms.

Cardiologist Peter Nixon coined the term 'people poisoning' to describe the stress induced by daily confrontation with hundreds, perhaps thousands, of total strangers. In many ways the process is directly analogous to the overload induced in the immune system by having to confront great numbers of strange molecules: we have to assess and classify every other person we encounter.

The stress of confronting all these strangers is compounded by the social stresses that abound in our everyday lives. We protect ourselves by building support structures of relationships which allow us to feel safe – only to be exposed to even higher levels of stress if these relationships fail, or we lose those we love. These emotional stresses generate reactions in our brains and hormone systems that can directly suppress immune reactions, or alternatively may keep our bodies constantly vigilant, exposing us to the hazard of overreaction and allergy. If we could maintain a constant level of happiness, our immune systems would function well, but this is a dream we can never quite achieve.

The crucial role of other people in immune disruption is in the maintenance of a culture that has the disruption of immunity built into many of its patterns of living. Social pressures cause people to adopt habits that damage immunity and cultural attitudes that lead people to value unnecessary commodities over their health.

Many people believe, erroneously, that we evolved in a jungle where almost everything was a threat to human life. Under such conditions life would have been intolerable, we would have given up and long ago become extinct. But today we have created such a jungle; all the things which we release into our environment to disrupt our immune system are threats to our lives more real than the snakes and tigers of our imaginary past. This new self-created jungle needs cutting back before it overwhelms us.

PART 2

DEALING
WITH DISEASE

We only feel we have to deal with disease when we become aware of symptoms. Until this happens everything is kept more or less under control by the immune system.

What we recognize as symptoms are, in the main, the results of the body's escalation of the war. Most of the body is in the same position as a town close to a battle zone. While it may not be directly involved in the fight, the battle draws in resources from its surroundings; parts of the body may be damaged by proximity to the action; and others may suffer from defensive measures, such as fever. No part of the body can be isolated from another, and symptoms of disease may be seen as a general rallying cry.

Our usual response is to turn to medicine. This is not always helpful or rational. For conditions where medicine has no answer the treatment may do more harm than good. Even where there is a specific treatment we should seek to understand why we succumb to the ailment and address that question rather than the symptoms. The defeat of the infectious scourges of the past was only achieved when causes were removed; medicine was not the primary weapon, rather it came along to mop up afterwards. Treating symptoms may make you feel better, but you should be aware of the circumstances when this could prolong your illness.

Symptoms of illness typically begin when interferons are holding up a pathogen, making us feel off colour for two or three days. After this time we may have produced sufficient antibodies and cloned enough lymphocytes to counter the threat, in which case we will have thrown it off. If not, specific symptoms will begin to emerge. We may develop a fever as the body makes the pathogens unwelcome, or develop spots or a coated tongue as debris accumulates from the battle zones.

We may lose weight as resources are converted to maintain the troops. Digestion and bowel functions may be affected as colonies of pathogens disrupt our supply and elimination systems. Headaches may occur with fever or as toxins build up.

At some point a crisis may occur and pass. Even though we begin to feel better, making good the war damage may take weeks or even months. We will feel weak from the depletion of local energy and material stores; lean tissue may have been recycled as well as fat. Many of the bacteria in our digestive system may have been wiped out; it will take time for them to re-establish numbers and balance, and while this is happening our metabolism will be working on limited inputs. We may suffer post-viral depression; we do not have a monopoly on chemical warfare, and many battle by-products can adversely affect our mood. In this state we become open to invasion by other pathogens. Pockets of the original pathogens may remain active long after the main war is over. If they adapt and evade the antibodies the whole cycle can begin again. Usually they linger on, fighting local rear-guard actions which may cause aches and pains, and leave us feeling under par. Eventually the surviving pathogens will give up and lie dormant, waiting to be passed on to someone else, or for our immune guard to drop.

When our battle with pathogens involves such astronomical numbers of troops and enemies the outcome is governed by the laws of probability. Pathogens and lymphocytes multiply exponentially. If lymphocytes increase at a faster rate than pathogens, we will win. In each case our chance of winning is governed by the probability that our immune defences will rise faster than the pathogens.

As we get older our metabolic processes tend to slow down. In addition, the capacity we have for producing appropriate populations of antibodies is progressively reduced. If a certain percentage remains committed to threats experienced in the past, it gives new attackers a head start in the race for our life, as a smaller percentage of antibodies is available for current threats. Both factors will reduce our response time, and the probability of success.

It is because these are the final limiting factors in dealing with disease that all the factors we have discussed in Part 1 are so important. In the chapters which follow we will discuss specific conditions and means of dealing with them as efficiently as possible.

Childhood Infections

The familiar diseases of childhood – chicken-pox, mumps, measles, and the like – result from virus infections. These are airborne viruses which arrive in epidemic waves. Having met them in childhood, most adults are immune to them, but those who lack specific immunity will develop an illness whose severity is determined by the general resilience of their immune systems.

Before birth, babies develop some background immunity to infections which are commonplace in their parents' society. The close links between the mother's circulation and that of her child mean that the baby can both suffer the mother's illness, if she is infected during pregnancy, and develop limited resistance to the pathogens to which she is immune. This background immunity moderates the effects of the diseases to which the child is likely to be exposed; without it, infections that we regard as mild can become life-threatening. New diseases have disproportionate effects on populations with no experience of them.

Breast-feeding reinforces the baby's immune defences. The colostrum in human milk contains immunoglobulins, proteins that confer immunity from the mother to her child. The absence of human colostrum from other types of infant feed is an important reason for the greater vulnerability to immune breakdown shown by bottle-fed babies.

However, disturbing recent research has revealed that human milk can be so contaminated with chemicals – such as pesticide residues – that it can actually damage babies. Mothers whose own bodies are heavily loaded with such chemicals can feed their babies more than the maximum doses fixed by the World Health Organization for adults. The consequences can be seen in the rising rate of eczema and similar allergic illness. Some of the traditional protective effects of breast-feeding are disappearing, while the prevalence and severity of allergies are increasing rapidly.

In view of the importance of breast milk to immunity, it is now imperative that prospective mothers should first improve the quality of their own flesh before bearing children. Adopting an organic wholefood diet and the other recommendations described in Chapter 2 a year before you plan to get pregnant will have this effect. Every mother-to-be should continue to eat an adequate organic and largely vegetarian diet during pregnancy and then throughout six months of breast-feeding in order to minimize intake of toxic chemicals and maximize her body's capacity to deal with them. This will mean that the milk she produces will tend to enhance, not damage, her baby's immunity.

In the first years of life, nearly all children go down with a series of minor ailments. Many will suffer half-a-dozen colds a year until their bodies become more familiar with rhinoviruses and susceptibility diminishes. Parts of their immune system may show the effects of this repeated attack. The tonsils, for example, may seem swollen for much of the time. Observing this link between swollen tonsils and colds led doctors and parents to imagine that the tonsils were themselves the source of the problem, not the body's way of dealing with infection. Consequently, millions of children have been subjected to unnecessary and painful tonsillectomies.

The healthy children of well-nourished mothers will have resilient immune systems capable of managing the infections they encounter, while the combination of poor nutrition with the irrational fashion for dieting during pregnancy, smoking, drug use and bottle-feeding produces vulnerable children. They are the ones who may become seriously ill if they encounter certain of our common infections.

Each whooping cough epidemic in Britain causes the death or long-term disablement of some very young children, often too young for vaccination. Our doctors and government spokespeople push vaccination as the only answer, yet in more affluent countries such as Sweden where poverty is effectively non-existent, there has not been a whooping cough death for decades. This is not because the disease has been eradicated through universal vaccination; quite the reverse. The Swedish authorities decided that the whooping cough vaccine was far too dangerous to recommend, and it is not generally used there. The difference between the whooping cough experiences of Sweden and Britain is due to the social differences between these countries.

A similar situation exists with measles. Improved living standards have produced a tremendous decline in the severity of measles in Britain. At the turn of the century, measles mortality was 318 per million of the population; in 1985, nine children died of measles. In poor Third World countries today, measles still kills millions, with an epidemic mortality rate which often reaches 25 per cent.

A healthy immune system is the key to resisting childhood epidemics. The first requirement is adequate nutrition; growing children should never be short of nutrient-rich food. It is indeed unfortunate that so much of the over-sweetened and processed junk-food produced today is made particularly attractive to children, many of whom will happily substitute useless or hazardous sugar and chemicals for the food they need. The role of vaccination is unquestionably secondary to that of nutrition. As the Swedish experience shows, British children do not die of whooping cough because they have not been vaccinated, but because impoverished living conditions among the disadvantaged sustain a more virulent infection. The same principle holds true for all types of disease.

Most childhood diseases are a part of our normal environment. Children should be kept healthy so that they may experience them and gain natural immunity.

6

Colds, 'Flu and
Other Respiratory
Infections

Causes

Almost all respiratory infections are caused by airborne viruses carried from
one person to another in tiny droplets of water in expired air. Occasionally,
viral infection so damages the membranes of the throat, ears or lungs that a
secondary bacterial infection will set in; but this is relatively rare and can be
avoided by appropriate action at the first signs of illness.

The ubiquitous common cold can be due to one of hundreds of rhinoviruses which, although sufficiently similar to cause the same pattern of
symptoms, differ enough to ensure that the antibodies developed in response
to a previous infection will not provide much protection against the next.
Cold viruses simply colonize the surface of the upper respiratory membranes,
the nose, throat and sinuses.

Influenza viruses are similar in many ways to rhinoviruses, though there
are fewer forms and they cause more severe symptoms. While each major
epidemic is usually due to a particular strain, two or three different strains
may be around at any time.

As infection attacks the membranes lower down the respiratory tract, it
can cause sore throat, loss of voice, bronchitis and pneumonia. These condi-

tions are usually due to viruses. In a minority of cases bacteria are involved, perhaps as secondary infections which build on damage caused by the initial viral infection; and other organisms such as *Pneumocystis carinii*, a single-celled creature, can attack the lungs of individuals whose immune systems have been weakened by AIDS or immunosuppressant drugs.

Acute attacks of bronchitis, an inflammation of the bronchial tubes that direct air into the lungs, usually have several interacting causes. *Ninety-five per cent* of people who suffer from bronchitis are smokers. Their respiratory membranes are particularly vulnerable to bacterial attack because of damage caused by smoking.

Symptoms

Respiratory infections usually begin with itchiness in the affected membranes. An itchy nose may make you sneeze — often the first symptom of attack by cold viruses. Itching in the throat or bronchi will make you cough, as the body tries to expel the cause of the irritation. The itching is a sign that the mast cells lining your respiratory membranes have been triggered by an invader, and are beginning to burst, releasing chemicals which cause inflammation and draw white cells to the battle zone. Pyrogens, temperature-elevating chemicals, are also released in the area, producing a heating sensation. Damaged cells produce *kinins*, which induce pain in the afflicted area. And mucus production increases to flush out unwanted organisms and cell debris.

Interferons will be produced to protect vulnerable cells from virus attack. High levels of interferon will make you feel unwell; depression and aches are characteristic side-effects of interferons. It is impossible to discriminate precisely between the effects of all the various disease-fighting chemicals as they spread into the body. Both pyrogens and interferons tend to induce fever. A higher temperature helps the body against the infection. This in turn can affect the brain, causing weakness, confusion, headache and even delirium. Your whole metabolic rate may speed up as your body gets into gear to fight the infection; your liver may release sugar so you do not feel hungry.

Different infections, of course, produce different patterns of effects, but the symptoms described above are due entirely to the body's effort to fight off the invaders. The actual damage inflicted by the virus may be imperceptible, though we can be sure that it would become all too obvious if the immune system's defences were to fail.

Outcome

Most battles with respiratory viruses are over before we know about them. The combined defences of the mucus layer, the immunoglobulins it contains and the mast cells with their selective elimination programmes prevent most infections from getting a hold.

Most respiratory infections are quite short-lived, especially if you do not interfere with the body's defences by using medicines to reduce symptoms. A cold may come and go in a couple of days; with 'flu, the acute phase of fever and aches will usually last for about three days, but it can be a week or more before health and energy return. Unfortunately, the damage caused by an infection and the body's response to it can sometimes be much longer-lasting. When emotional depression follows severe virus infection, it can last for weeks or months.

Both virus and bacterial respiratory infections can, on occasion, cause serious illness. In those whose immune systems are weak, 'flu or a severe cold may lead to pneumonia. 'Flu killed millions when people were malnourished and badly housed, and smoke from coal fires polluted the air of urban areas, damaging the respiratory membranes of all those exposed to it. It has been estimated that 20 million died in the 'flu pandemic of 1918. In 1985, 662 deaths due to influenza were recorded in England and Wales, and 27,931 due to pneumonia; almost all of these were among the elderly or bedridden.

Vectors

We catch respiratory infections by breathing air containing viruses. Obviously, the more people who breathe the same air over short periods of time, the more pathogens they are likely to encounter. Coughs, colds, 'flu and the less common respiratory ailments are most common among urban populations, especially those working with many others inside closed buildings.

Ideal conditions for the spread of respiratory infection are provided by air conditioning and central heating, combined with energy-efficient buildings without currents of fresh air or windows which open. Our crowded cities,

86

providing close contact between millions of people, ensure that huge numbers swap viruses on a day-to-day basis. We have a work ethic that makes matters even better for pathogens and worse for people: we encourage people to take their viruses into the office to share with colleagues, rather than keeping them at home where their spread would be somewhat limited. Consequently, each new form of rhinovirus produces a minor epidemic, afflicting millions. While we are able to develop resistance to successive variations on the cold theme, we do not seem to find it necessary to question a way of life that inevitably subjects most adults to two or three colds a year, and children, too young to have a complete library of antibodies, to colds every other month.

Postive Action

Increased vulnerability to respiratory infections is associated with damage to the respiratory membranes and immune incompetence. Positive action to enhance immunity needs to be directed both at ensuring the effectiveness of the membrane protective systems and at improving the general immune status of the body.

Reducing Susceptibility

The specific comments below complement the general immune enhancement that will result from changing your lifestyle in accordance with the recommendations made in Chapter 2.

Avoid polluted air: Building up defences against respiratory viruses requires that the membranes should be allowed to function without any hindrance. The most important action is to avoid air pollution – particularly cigarette smoke.

A careful study comparing a group of young people who smoked cigarettes with a matched group of non-smokers during a 'flu epidemic revealed that the majority of non-smokers avoided infection completely. Among those non-smokers who did develop 'flu symptoms, the illness was not severe. By contrast, the smokers were twice as likely to go down with 'flu, and all those who became seriously ill were smokers.

In general, the more you are exposed to smoke – whether from your own

87

cigarettes or someone else's – the greater your vulnerability to colds, 'flu, bronchitis and other respiratory infections.

Avoid excessively dry air: Although damp housing has been convincingly linked with an increased risk of bronchitis, in this age of central heating excessively dry air is now more of a problem for many people. Dry air can dehydrate the mucous coating of the nostrils so that its effectiveness is reduced and viruses are able to penetrate more easily. So if you are prone to colds and you live or work in a dry atmosphere, invest in a humidifier. One study in Canada revealed that the use of humidifiers in schools reduced absenteeism by 40 per cent; other research has confirmed this effect, although the degree of benefit detected does vary from study to study.

It is widely believed that damp – especially from a ducking or damp feet – makes people more prone to coughs and colds. This could be because a lower temperature helps the viruses, and being chilled when you are already fighting a virus adds to the stress on your body and therefore may reduce your resistance. Research has confirmed that people who are exposed to cold when cold viruses are incubating in their bodies are more likely to develop symptoms of infection.

Increase vitamin C intake: Vitamin C is a crucial nutrient for protection from virus infection, and it seems to be particularly important both in reducing susceptibility to colds and in limiting the effects of infection. Those whose everyday diet provides plentiful vitamin C are less likely to catch colds, and large doses of the vitamin at the first sign of viral attack can prevent it from taking hold.

We believe it is not wise to take mega-doses of vitamin C on a daily basis. This is because the synthetic vitamin can irritate the digestive tract, and because this sort of approach can disrupt the complex metabolic balance of the body. It is much more sensible to take nutrients in the form of good food, and use mega-doses very rarely, and then only if you do not suffer adverse effects such as diarrhoea.

Dietary vitamin C can be scarce in the winter months and early spring. This may explain the prevalence of colds at this time of year. The vitamin disappears gradually when food is stored, and more rapidly with cooking and processing. The answer is to eat plenty of whole citrus fruit and to grow beansprouts on your kitchen windowsill. Eat beansprouts fresh in salads and sandwiches for their remarkable nutrient content.

When you feel the first signs of respiratory infection, increase your intake of citrus to the equivalent of half-a-dozen oranges a day. Maintain this level of intake for four days. This will enhance absorption of dietary zinc as well as delivering vitamin C and useful bioflavinoids.

Activity: At the first sign of infection, rest! Do not stress your body with any strenuous activity. Your energy is needed to fight the infection. In particular, avoid vigorous activity in cold air, for the chill will help the virus and hinder your body's efforts.

Medicines

There are a great many proprietory cough, cold and 'flu remedies on the market, and most people will take these and/or aspirin or paracetamol to help them cope with the unpleasant symptoms of infection. In terms of enhancing the immune response, taking such medicines is almost always irrational and counter-productive. These symptoms are produced by the immune system and, by suppressing them, you suppress the fight against the virus. So do not take any medicine for your cold; just keep warm, take things easy, and eat well.

89

If you want something to make you feel better, it should do no harm. Warm drinks will help your body. Hot water with honey and lemon is excellent; a hot toddy may cheer you, but do not drink so much alcohol that you stress your liver.

It is especially important that you drink more than usual when you have a fever, as in 'flu. You need extra liquid to counterbalance the sweating caused by the fever and to help your body flush out the debris of infection. Herb teas or lemon and honey mixtures are best.

In more serious bacterial or parasitic respiratory infections, your body may require help. Your doctor will prescribe antibiotics if he has good reason to believe that the infection is not caused by a virus — but such infections are relatively rare. There is nothing that medicine can do to help your body in the fight against respiratory viruses.

Tonsillectomy and Other Types of Surgery

Recurrent colds and sore throats in childhood have inspired the introduction of a range of potentially and actually harmful treatments. The most dramatically dangerous of these was the American fad for irradiation of the

IMMUNITY PLUS

thymus, described in Chapter 4, but British surgeons have also caused widespread damage by removing parts of the immune system which would have provided life-long protection against respiratory infection.

Tonsillectomy used to be a routine operation for millions of children. Frequently, the adenoids were removed too. Some surgeons are still doing this. Yet such surgery causes irreparable damage to the immune system, for these organs produce white blood cells and antibodies against infection in the throat. Although the lymph glands in the neck seem to be able to take over the function of the lost tonsils and adenoids, there will be some loss of effectiveness.

Vaccination

Vaccines have been developed against both colds and 'flu but their value is limited. With over a hundred variations on the common cold theme, the prospects of a useful vaccine are very remote; but since each 'flu epidemic may involve just a few variants, a carefully aimed vaccine can help vulnerable people to escape it. 'Flu vaccination is used on a limited scale, and your doctor may recommend it for you if there is reason to believe that you would suffer a particularly severe illness if you were to catch 'flu.

There is a slight risk associated with 'flu vaccination, so it does not make sense to vaccinate everyone against every variety of 'flu virus. For most of us, it is enough to behave in such a way that we keep our resistance high.

Limiting the Spread of Respiratory Infections

Colds are probably more prevalent today than they have ever been. There are two main reasons for this. Firstly, we are crowded into cities in larger numbers and larger working units than ever before. Secondly, most people are very casual about respiratory infections, so they go about their business as usual, ignoring or suppressing the unpleasant symptoms.

During the last war, the government propaganda machine pushed the message 'Coughs and sneezes spread diseases'. True enough – but their response ('Trap the germs in your handkerchief') would not prevent their spread any more effectively than today's cold treatments. To limit the spread of these infections and reduce the misery they cause, we need to take them much more seriously, refusing to go to work or school or associate with other people while we are infectious. Employers should encourage this sort of behaviour, not discourage it as most do today. In the long run, over-zealous individuals are not good for corporate health. Perhaps the spread of more serious airborne infections will force us to be less casual about viruses.

Salmonella
and the Stomach
Bugs

Causes

Many intestinal infections are caused by viruses. The enteroviruses are the
gut equivalents of the rhinoviruses that cause colds; the old-fashioned idea
of 'a cold on the tummy' is actually quite accurate. These common infections
produce short-lived symptoms that are rarely severe in healthy people.
More serious or more persistent infections may be caused by other types of
pathogens: bacteria, such as salmonella and shingella, which are responsible
for food poisoning and dysentery; fungi, notably candida; single-celled
creatures including amoebae; and intestinal worms of various kinds.

Organisms that colonize the gut generally arrive on or in our food and
drink. Infections are most often spread by poor food, hygiene, storage or
cooking practices, although some can be carried by flies, notably the
housefly. Public health measures have done much to prevent the delivery of
such pathogens to our tables, but recent developments are changing the
situation. Dominant among these are changes in farming practice which
have produced an increase in the prevalence of bacterial infection. The
extensive use of antibiotics for livestock has produced super-strains of
bacteria which are resistant to drug treatment.

Bacterial Infection (Food Poisoning) – Symptoms

Symptoms can take anything from one hour to eight days to develop, depending on the pathogen involved, the resistance of the victim and the number of organisms consumed. The usual timescale is between twelve and twenty-four hours.

Acute intestinal infections all produce the same general symptom pattern. The gut becomes distended and painful (tummy-ache); there is usually nausea and often vomiting, and copious watery diarrhoea. Fever, weakness and headache are also quite common.

The pathogens that attack the gut typically produce toxins that enter the body through the intestinal wall. The immune system responds by flooding the area with water and chemical products from the mast cells lining the intestine. This reaction produces inflammation with associated discomfort (gastro-enteritis), and draws more defensive cells to the area. Diarrhoea is a very understandable reaction by the body; it ensures rapid and thorough elimination of as many pathogens and associated toxins as possible in the shortest period of time.

Usually the whole episode is over in a period of a few hours, perhaps a day – though the diarrhoea may linger – and the consequences are rarely serious. Nevertheless, such infections can be dangerous to those whose resistance is low, particularly the elderly, the sick and underweight babies.

93

Incidence

Intestinal infections are common, but most episodes are never reported and do not appear in statistics on food poisoning. However, the available statistics reveal that the incidence of such infections has been increasing, and that they occur most often in the second half of the year – in late summer and autumn. Notification levels hovered between 5,000 and 8,000 in the mid sixties; by 1975 they were over 11,000, and they have remained at this higher level since.

The recorded outbreaks are predominantly the larger-scale ones that get investigated by public health laboratories. Hospitals are often involved. Ironically, food poisoning in a hospital is likely to have particularly serious consequences. If the organisms concerned originate in the hospital they are likely to be antibiotic-resistant and may be especially virulent. The patients who are then exposed to them will be less able to resist the illness caused. A hospital outbreak of salmonella or staphylococcal food poisoning can lead to several deaths.

With the advent of sophisticated food preservation and cooking methods and almost universal refrigerator ownership, food poisoning should be on the decline. That it is not is likely to be due to the increased consumption of intensively reared poultry and factory-farmed pigs and other meat animals. These unfortunate creatures are kept in conditions of such overcrowding that infections are endemic. Farmers have responded by routinely giving animals antibiotics. The effect has been to breed salmonellae and other bacteria, capable of causing quite severe illness in humans, that show multiple resistance to our most important antibiotics.

Antibiotic-resistant strains spread from the intestines of these animals to people. Here, previously relatively benign organisms can pick up new genetic material which transforms them into drug-resistant strains. So as they move from animal to man, and from one person to another, these bacteria become more dangerous.

Freezing merely slows bacteria down. They can be killed by heat, but they can survive low-temperature roasting or stewing, and they multiply in cooked meat at a rate which is dependent on temperature. So a piece of rare meat, or a cooked meat dish eaten a day or so after preparation, may contain millions of these organisms. Re-heated food will not be sterilized unless the temperature is well above the normal boiling point of water. Pressure-cooking can destroy bacteria; warming-up will not – it may merely speed multiplication.

Prepared meat dishes such as pies and sausages can often harbour salmonellae. In one study reported in the *Journal of Hygiene*, 413 of 854 packets of pork sausages from one large manufacturer were positive for salmonella. On average, 30 per cent of packs of sausages and sausage meat from various sources were contaminated with these bacteria – sometimes many types in the same pack.

After meat, milk products and fried rice are the next most important sources of food poisoning. Boiled rice is very rarely a problem, but fried rice is usually pre-cooked, left to stand for an indefinite period, and re-heated in fat, so any bacteria have a good opportunity to multiply. Shellfish can be hazardous, particularly oysters which are eaten raw, for many grow in sewage-rich estuaries where they pick up pathogens excreted by local people.

Vegetables – especially fresh vegetables – rarely cause problems, because they do not provide good culture media for pathogenic organisms. So even raw vegetables grown organically, using manure or bone meal which could be contaminated, will tend to be safe. Nevertheless, it is always wise to wash vegetables thoroughly before eating them.

For many of us, intestinal infections only cause problems when we go abroad. It used to be assumed by chauvinists that foreign meant dirty, that other countries' water was not as good as ours, and so on. Unprejudiced experience reveals that the problem is more one of exposure to a different microscopic ecosystem, one to which our own immune systems are not accustomed.

Positive Action

Food hygiene is obviously important to avoid large-scale outbreaks of intestinal infections. Legal controls and regular inspection of kitchens are clearly not enough to protect us from these diseases. Farming practice should be reformed on the grounds of health alone; animals reared in conditions that are conducive to health do not need antibiotics and do not become breeding-grounds for drug-resistant and super-virulent pathogens. The moral argument against the cruelty of factory farming merely adds strength and urgency to the case. Demanding naturally reared meat and poultry from free-range animals will protect you and add to the economic pressure that will eventually persuade farmers to change.

The immune competence of the gut membrane is undoubtedly reduced by processed twentieth-century food and drink. Chlorine and chlorine compounds in our water may kill the bacteria in the water supply but they can also damage the intestine. So an efficient purifying system that removes chlorine from your cooking and drinking water is a must. Pure bottled water for drinking also makes sense.

The most dramatic evidence for the importance of good immune function in protection from intestinal infection was a demonstration by scientist and social reformer, Max von Pettenkofer. He claimed that he could bring cholera under control in Munich by ensuring that the city had a supply of pure water which was kept free of contamination by sewage. The dramatic decrease in the incidence of cholera proved him correct. But Pettenkofer did not accept that the presence of the cholera bacillus was the only factor that mattered in infection. To prove his point, he obtained a culture of cholera bacilli from its discoverer, Robert Koch. These organisms had come from a person who had recently died of cholera in Hamburg. Pettenkofer confidently swallowed the bacilli. Huge numbers were found in his stools, yet the only illness he suffered was a mild diarrhoea, and fellow-workers who tried the same experiment also came to no harm.

Reducing the Severity of Infection

If you fall victim to intestinal infection, the most important action you can take is to drink plenty of pure water. Aim for six pints in twenty-four hours. Dehydration is the most serious consequence of intestinal infection, and rehydration has been shown to be highly effective in saving the lives of vulnerable people. If the sufferer is a baby or an elderly person, it is wise to add honey and a small pinch each of bicarbonate and salt to the water. Rehydration salts are also available from chemists' shops. Avoid all other food and drink for twenty-four hours and gradually reintroduce it when the symptoms have abated.

Medicine

Most forms of medication for diarrhoea contain drugs which suppress the symptom at the cost of extending the course of the illness. Diarrhoea serves a valuable function. Such palliatives as kaolin and morph and other remedies, both traditional and new, should therefore be avoided completely. Antibiotics are usually useless for these infections, and they can make the problem worse by disrupting the gut flora. Most doctors now know better than to prescribe them except for lasting attacks of diarrhoea when the pathogen has been identified and responds to antibiotic therapy.

Fungal Infestations of the Gut – Causes

It has become fashionable in some alternative medical circles to blame a whole host of intestinal problems on *Candida albicans* (thrush), the yeast that is most familiar as the cause of an itchy inflammation of the vagina. It is not yet clear how common or serious the problem actually is, but the frequency of invasive thrush infections among AIDS patients and other immune-compromised people makes it clear that this is a condition associated with immune depression.

Candida is a normal inhabitant of the healthy bowel, but under certain circumstances it grows out of control and invades membranes. This may happen because reduced immunity interferes with the body's protective systems, so that the fungus can penetrate more readily. Or it may happen when an individual takes antibiotics which selectively kill bacteria and thus reduce the competition which normally limits the proliferation of fungi. It is possible that there is a genuine and largely unrecognized epidemic of thrush infestation of the gut affecting many members of the population. Diabetics and women who take oral contraceptives are particularly at risk.

Two main factors lead us to suspect that there is a real thrush epidemic. Firstly, the continual use of antibiotics and hormones in animal feed means that consuming meat and eggs produced by factory-farming methods will give low levels of these drugs on a daily basis. The internal ecology is bound to be affected, with the yeasts gaining an advantage relative to bacteria. Secondly, the chronic immune depression that is a product of the processed diet and Western lifestyle will further reduce resistance to candida. The frequency with which many women are afflicted with vaginal thrush adds weight to this argument.

97

Symptoms

An overgrowth of *Candida albicans* is believed to be responsible for many cases of food intolerance, allergies, indigestion and emotional symptoms. At one end of the digestive tract, it can be seen as white patches on the tongue and throat; at the other, it causes anal itching. Chronic thrush infection of the gut is usually associated with recurring or incurable vaginal thrush. The presence of the fungus can be confirmed by cultured smears taken from the affected parts.

Positive Action

Since *Candida albicans* is to be found in all of us, there is no sense in attempting to avoid catching it. We must maintain our bodies in a state of healthy balance so that the fungus does not proliferate.

Diet

Candida sufferers should avoid any source of antibiotics. Meat and poultry should not be eaten, unless it can be guaranteed drug-free. Eggs must always be free-range.

Live yoghurt is particularly valuable for rebalancing the gut flora. It contains *Lactobacillus acidophilus* (also found in human milk), a beneficial bacterium which competes with potentially harmful organisms and produces mildly acid conditions in the bowel. When the environment is slightly acid, candida does not proliferate. Always choose natural live yoghurt, not the mass-produced preservative-rich flavoured varieties.

Even if you are intolerant of milk, you are likely to be able to enjoy yoghurt safely. The lactobacillus digests the milk sugars which are the usual cause of milk intolerance. However, you may prefer sheep's or goat's milk yoghurt.

Lactobacillus acidophilus can be obtained from some health shops to be consumed as a dry culture. Bear in mind, however, that this bacterium thrives on milk products, and is not likely to thrive in your body unless it receives the nourishment it requires; if you dislike yoghurt, take lactobacillus with Camembert cheese, which contains other anti-thrush nutrients. Half a litre a day of live natural yoghurt should quickly rebalance the bowel. Maintain your lactobacillus population by making live yoghurt part of your normal everyday diet.

At the same time, you should increase your intake of both biotin and oleic acid. A particularly rich source of biotin is free-range eggs, but eggs must always be cooked; eating raw or undercooked eggs can cause biotin deficiency. Oleic acid is found in olive oil; use plenty of cold-pressed olive oil in your salad dressings. Avocado vinaigrette is a particularly tasty anti-thrush food, rich in biotin, folic acid, vitamin B6, vitamin E and oleic acid!

The ravages of candida will require high levels of healing nutrients — particularly vitamins E and B6 and zinc — nutrients that are in very short supply in the normal Western diet. An organic wholefood diet should contain all you need.

It is said by some US doctors that a diet which contains yeasts or fermented products encourages the growth of candida. We have seen no convincing evidence of this, nor does it seem to have biological plausibility; baking and brewing yeasts are not the same as candida and do not colonize the human body. We do not therefore believe that it is necessary to give up bread and other yeasted foods in order to overcome candida; however, further evidence on this point may emerge in the future.

Medicine

Anti-fungal drugs, particularly nystatin tablets, are prescribed for candida sufferers. These can be very useful in the short term, but unless other action is taken to rebuild immunity and rebalance the gut flora, they are often ineffective in the longer term and the infection soon recurs. In due course, candida is liable to become resistant to the popular fungicides; some strains are already showing resistance. Candida sufferers should avoid antibiotic therapy.

Other Intestinal Infestations

Small animals — worms, microscopic flagellates and protozoa — are the final group of organisms that can colonize the gut. Illness due to these creatures is uncommon in Britain. When they do occur, they are likely to be long-term parasites, producing relatively few distinct symptoms. More dangerous parasites are currently of little importance in the developed world.

The lining of the intestine has evolved defences against parasites. The immunoglobulins (IgE) which are involved in food allergy are primarily concerned with protecting us from worms and similar large parasites; when they work as intended, they are capable of causing severe damage to these unwanted organisms.

Two types of parasite have been causing increasingly common problems, particularly among gay men. One is the protozoon which causes amoebic dysentery; it is estimated that it now infects about 5 per cent of the US population. The other is the flagellate *Giardia lamblia*, discovered in 13.3 per cent of Scottish schoolchildren in a 1977 survey. Both cause intermittent diarrhoea, abdominal discomfort, and flatulence. Other symptoms can include nausea, weight loss, weakness and blood or pus in the faeces.

Avoiding Action

Organisms that infect the gut are transmitted through contact with faecal material. This is why it is important to wash your hands after using the lavatory. Indirect contact can occur through touching food with unwashed hands which carry pathogens, or through pathogens surviving on lavatory handles or shared towels, or even, perhaps, through children's play in contaminated sand-pits. Direct transmission occurs through kissing or licking the anus (analingus); this practice has been particularly widespread among male homosexuals and it is responsible for the spread of a variety of infections.

When drinking water is contaminated with sewerage, a wide range of pathogens can be spread into the population. Our sewers were built in Victorian times; today, in many parts of the country, they are disintegrating. Any leakage into the drinking water system is likely to result in local epidemics of diseases ranging from hepatitis to shingella.

While it is obviously sensible to take care with personal hygiene and to ensure that our children always wash their hands thoroughly after using the lavatory or even just flushing it, it remains true that our intestinal immune systems are capable of protecting us from small numbers of pathogens that arrive with food and water, or when we suck our thumbs or chew our fingernails. If this were not the case, we should all have succumbed as children to the many pathogens that abound in the environment. So we return, once more, to the crucial importance of maintaining our individual immune systems in a high state of readiness to deal with all potential problems.

To maintain the integrity of the immune systems of the gut, diet and quality of water are particularly crucial. We must eat the sort of food on which our bodies and our intestines work best – the balanced organic wholefood diet described in Chapter 2. This alone may be sufficient to protect us from intestinal disease, but we cannot afford to confuse our immune defences with strange chemicals, or strip away our beneficial bacteria with chlorine and antibiotics. We should aim never to disturb our internal environment with laxatives or enemas; with the correct diet, these are unnecessary.

Close Contact
Diseases

In this and the following two chapters we shall be discussing diseases which are transmitted by close contact between people. Although the most common mode of transmission involves sexual acts, this is not necessarily the case with all such diseases. If you are concerned about AIDS you should read this and the following chapter.

By concentrating on the sexual aspect of transmission we have put many conditions into a stigmatized class. The shame, confusion, and hypocrisy which surrounds sexuality in our culture has helped drive these diseases underground. Our attitudes help these diseases survive, to the detriment of us all.

Close contact diseases (CCDs) can be transmitted in any intimate relationship between people. Such situations include contact between mother and baby during pregnancy and after birth; kissing, fighting and biting between children, or between lovers; any sexual act involving penetration of a body orifice by a part of another's body. To a lesser degree, the sharing of penetrative objects; the government's AIDS warning noted toothbrushes, but illogically omitted sex toys such as dildoes and vibrators. Blood-to-blood contact offers another vector for CCDs; needles, in dentistry, tattooing and drug addiction, are a possible source if not adequately sterilized; blood or blood-product transfusions are another; fighting, where knuckles split on tooth and lip, could offer another. At the extreme, sharing anything contaminated with body fluids from another person poses some degree of risk.

Pregnancy is a special situation where the mother's blood circulation is connected with her baby's, and infectious organisms carried in the blood (such as AIDS, hepatitis and syphilis) can be passed to the baby. Localized infections of the genital tract can be transmitted during birth. Unfortunately, pregnancy also involves immune suppression in the mother's body, so that her immune system does not reject the baby; this can mean that infections originally transmitted to the mother by close contact with other adults can flare up during pregnancy and may be transmitted to the baby. It is therefore particularly important that any prospective mother is careful to avoid infection.

Causes

A variety of organisms from all groups can be transmitted by close contact. Such contact allows the direct transfer of pathogens from a suitable environment in or on one person to a similar situation in or on another. The most delicate organisms can be transferred in bodily fluids in this way; they travel with their environment, thus evading some of our defences.

CCDs due to bacteria include: syphilis, gonorrhea, and non-specific urethritis (NSU). Those due to viruses include: infectious mononucleosis (glandular fever, often called 'the kissing disease' because of its mode of transmission), herpes, hepatitis, warts and AIDS. Infections due to micro-organisms include trichomonas and chlamydia. Fungi can cause athlete's foot, ringworm, and genital candida (thrush).

Transmission

CCDs are usually spread in infected bodily fluids, such as semen, saliva, vaginal secretions and secretions produced by sores or lesions the condition may generate. Fungi and warts can spread by direct skin-to-skin contact.

Sharing bodily fluids with another is vital for the continuation of life, but it is always risky. It means sharing many of the pathogens to which the other person has been exposed. Aside from breeding, without intimate contact with others we fail to thrive individually. Some may be able to divert the needs and energy involved into a spiritual cause, but for most isolation makes us vulnerable to other forms of ill-health.

We have to limit our contact with others to reduce the risk of CCDs. Naturally the risks are least when intimacy is restricted to the immediate circle of family. Until recently many of us felt we could be quite casual in our contact with other people; the heady days of sexual freedom hid the resurgence of viral infections. AIDS has brought a rough awakening; now we have to regard all other people as potential sources of serious infection.

For adults this means that acting to avoid AIDS will protect from the other serious CCDs. Fortunately those conditions which are likely to predominate in other intimate situations are amenable to treatment or defeat by the immune system.

Symptoms

CCDs can produce many different symptoms. With some they are localized in the genital organs and specific to the infection. Sores or lesions around bodily orifices are common symptoms of viral or bacterial infection, but women may not be aware of internal symptoms such as warts. If any of their previous partners have such symptoms, they should go to the local STD (sexually transmitted disease) clinic for a check-up. Itching is characteristic of fungal infestations. Unusual discharges may indicate genital infection; these should be checked out promptly at the STD clinic.

103

Most viral CCDs are capable of producing symptoms such as fever and general malaise, which affect the whole body; they may cause no symptoms at all at the point of contact. Their time-course is very variable; some have phases of varying duration, interrupted by latent periods of varying length. Definite diagnosis usually requires a blood test.

Prognosis

CCDs can linger on for long periods, bouncing back and forth among the same group of people indefinitely. The greatest problem they pose is that they are *intimate* with us, both in transmission, and in their integration with our bodily processes.

For both reasons it is important to take this group of diseases very seriously and do whatever is necessary to limit their spread to others. Anyone who has a CCD must contain it to themselves. This means restricting your contact with others, not becoming pregnant, or indulging in any affectionate or sexual act which allows the infection to spread. Specialist advice and treatment may also be necessary.

9

AIDS

AIDS is an acronym for Acquired Immune Deficiency Syndrome. AIDS is not a single disease but a pattern of illness, now known to be the final stage of infection by the Human Immunodeficiency Virus (HIV). The syndrome develops late in a continuous sequence of events and its precise form varies widely between individuals, so a precise definition of what constitutes AIDS has proved elusive. AIDS is now diagnosed in patients who develop diseases which suggest a severe underlying cellular immune deficiency in the absence of any known cause of reduced resistance, and the HIV virus or antibodies to it are found in the blood.

The syndrome was first recognized in 1981, when young men in San Francisco and New York were found to be suffering from diseases which had only previously been seen among people whose immune systems were severely suppressed, usually by drugs prescribed to prevent rejection of transplants. As the numbers of cases grew, it became apparent that the cause was likely to be a new type of virus. Within three years, three independent laboratories had isolated a new virus from the blood of sufferers. Groups of scientists gave the virus different names: LAV was used by France's Institut Pasteur, in the United States it was called HTLV-III; other names included IDAV and ARV. Eventually, the scientific and medical community agreed to name the virus HIV (Human Immunodeficiency Virus).

HIV is an unusual sort of virus, a *retrovirus*. This means that in place of

DNA (deoxyribonucleic acid), the genetic material that most viruses contain, HIV relies on a different form, RNA (ribonucleic acid). Using a special enzyme (reverse transcriptase: its existence is inferred from its effects, from which its name was derived), retroviruses create DNA from their RNA. This means that there is an extra step in their replication.

Perhaps as a consequence of this extra step, HIV is remarkably unstable, changing as it reproduces. It changes its genetic nature and its antigens faster than any other known virus. Indeed, so rapid is this process that infected individuals have been found to have many variants of the virus, all of which have emerged during the course of infection. This adds to the problem that HIV causes to the immune system. It means that any antibodies that are produced will quickly cease to be effective. It poses tremendous problems for those who are trying to develop vaccines, and leads to problems in tests to detect the presence of the virus.

Many sub-forms of HIV have already emerged; there are two major varieties, classified as HIV-1 and HIV-2, which show only 40 per cent overlap in their genetic codes. The long-term results of this rapid evolution are unpredictable; the virus could die out or become more virulent.

Uncertainty remains about the time and place of origin of HIV. There is evidence that the virus was already infecting people in Africa as early as 1966. It probably evolved spontaneously in Africa from a similar virus which affects green monkeys. While it is possible that HIV evolved from the interaction of the green monkey virus and a sheep virus, scrapie, during laboratory experiments in which monkeys were infected with scrapie, we believe that natural evolution is much more likely. The disease has spread far more widely and rapidly in Africa than among people associated with biological research establishments in the developed world.

HIV infection is spread in body fluids, most often through sex, contaminated needles, and blood or blood products. Although the threat it poses to the human species is deeply alarming, we should not forget that most of us can avoid infection quite easily. We need not be exposed to dirty needles and we can adapt our sexual behaviour to minimize the risk of catching or spreading infection. Already, behaviour changes among some of those most at risk appear to have been reflected in a fall in the rate at which HIV infection is spreading. We should not make the mistake of focussing so closely on the medical horrors of AIDS that we fail to acknowledge that dealing with this epidemic is a social and behavioural challenge which we can rise to meet.

The problem of AIDS is particularly tragic in Africa, where many different factors have contributed to the severity of the epidemic. One is the particular vulnerability of the African people to HIV, both because of their genetic make-up (a point to which we return below) and because of the patterns of social behaviour and attitudes which predominate in the worst-afflicted areas.

Another factor which some experts believe to be important is the campaign for the eradication of smallpox, which began in 1967. The incidence of AIDS in Africa mirrors the record of vaccination against smallpox, and it is possible that HIV could have been stimulated into virulence by the action of the smallpox vaccine. Experience in the United States has shown that routine vaccination with live vaccines like that used against smallpox can precipitate the development of AIDS in individuals who are harbouring HIV. Multiple use of needles in the anti-smallpox campaign could have added to the problem by spreading the virus. The re-use of needles for routine vaccinations and a general laxness about sterilization of sharp instruments used in both traditional and Western medicine is believed to be a major cause of AIDS among African children today.

Racial differences in susceptibility to HIV infection reflect differences in genetic characteristics between peoples of geographically diverse origins. There seems to be a link between the effectiveness of transport of vitamin D (derived from sunlight) and resistance to this virus, a link which favours pale-skinned people. Relatively few Caucasian people have the genetic make-up which makes them particularly vulnerable; while less that 1 per cent of the general British population show the genetic marker known as Gc 1f 1f, 30 per cent of AIDS patients have it. This genetic difference produces relative, not absolute, resistance to HIV infection. It implies that the course of the AIDS epidemic in Europe is likely to be less severe than in Africa.

There is mounting evidence that most healthy people have considerable resistance to HIV, while those whose immune systems have been compromised are particularly likely to succumb to the effects of the virus. Homosexuals and drug addicts developed AIDS first partly because their immunity had already been undermined by their lifestyle. People who have many sexual partners are exposed to all the viruses that their partners have encountered. In addition, exposure to the foreign proteins in sperm from many other people puts greater demand on the immune system, reducing immune competence. Drug addiction means that the metabolic processes which underwrite immunity are compromised. Heroin addicts suffer further

107

damage to immunity through loss of appetite and disinterest in food and most are severely undernourished. In addition, like some of the more promiscuous homosexuals who are at high risk of developing AIDS, drug addicts are liable to suffer from the debilitating effects of liver damage due to hepatitis B infection. For both groups the result is that HIV gets an easy ride.

Those who are already infected can, by understanding the nature of the virus and its action, reduce the severity of its effects. It is possible to remain healthy for many years despite HIV by taking deliberate and appropriate action to protect immunity, adopting behaviour patterns that tip the balance in favour of survival and against the proliferation of the virus.

Causes

The Human Immunodeficiency Virus attacks the immune system and the brain. It breeds inside white cells of the immune system and related cells of the brain, destroying them in the process. The cells it selects are those with a particular type of marker on their surface to which the virus is able to attach itself; this marker is most common on T-helper cells and Natural Killers, the very cells which should combat a viral invader. These cells are thus selectively damaged by HIV. One of the hallmarks of HIV infection is a fall in the number of T-helper cells.

Even before the infected cells are destroyed, the presence of the virus within them can incapacitate them, blinding them to the activities of pathogens against which they would otherwise mount a defence. Pathogens which are normally dealt with as a matter of routine can multiply unchecked and produce virulent forms of disease.

This can take many years. HIV is one of a small group of slow, or *lente* viruses, characterized by long delays in the disease processes they cause. The syndrome recognized as AIDS can take up to a decade and perhaps even longer to emerge, so nobody can make definitive statements about what proportion of infected people will eventually develop it. Sometimes any symptoms are mild and it is possible that serious disease may never develop; however it is too early to be sure of this. In other cases, HIV causes fatal illness which may not fit the accepted medical definition of AIDS.

Exposure to HIV does not necessarily lead to infection. It can be repulsed by healthy immune defences. However, there is a large element of uncertainty in any individual case, so exposure will always be risky even to the fittest person. Nobody, even those who seem to have high immunity to virus infection, can afford to be confident that they would be able to resist HIV. There are so many unknown factors that avoidance is the only safe option.

If HIV enters the bloodstream directly, through damaged membranes, shared needles, or contaminated blood transfusion, the virus has unimpeded access to white cells and the risk is greatly increased. Yet even then people vary widely in their susceptibility to its worst effects.

After a variable length of time, usually about three months but sometimes years, the body responds to HIV infection by producing antibodies. These have no apparent influence on the course of the disease but they are used as markers which can be detected in tests for HIV infection. Because of the delay in appearance of antibodies, there may be no evidence of infection when the virus is in fact present. This has meant that contaminated blood which carried the virus but not the marker antibody has evaded detection, and some people have become victims despite screening of donated blood. The problem may be resolved by the development of tests which detect the virus directly, but these are not yet in general use.

The detection problem is compounded by the existence of different forms of the virus and of antibodies to it. It is not always possible to detect HIV even in the blood of AIDS sufferers. The risk of receiving contaminated blood is nevertheless low in Western countries, but in Africa and Third World countries where AIDS is rife and screening facilities may be inadequate, blood transfusions are bound to carry a higher risk.

Antibody production is probably stimulated by relatively rapid replication of HIV. This occurs when white cells which harbour the virus react against other infections, activating HIV, which then proliferates. Consequently, any infection suffered by someone whose white cells have been invaded by HIV will lead to severe damage to the immune system. This makes them more vulnerable to further infection, accelerating the destruction. Eventually the capacity of certain sectors of immunity is so restricted that the system fails. At this point, multiple infections afflict the victim, and it is these, together with brain damage directly due to HIV, that cause death from AIDS.

Many of the infections that ravage AIDS patients can only succeed when the immune system is depressed. These are called 'opportunistic' infections;

they include a form of pneumonia due to *Pneumocystis carinii* which used to be unknown except among those whose immune systems were suppressed with drugs. The characteristic cancers found in AIDS patients are caused by viruses which do not produce severe consequences under any other circumstances; for example, Kaposi's sarcoma, the most common of these, is related to infection with cytomegalovirus, which often causes no symptoms at all in people with normal levels of immunity. Kaposi's sarcoma used to occur only as a superficial skin disease in men over the age of sixty but in AIDS victims it is strikingly aggressive, invading many organs, the purplish skin lesions representing only the surface evidence of extensive internal damage.

Other infections common in AIDS are familiar to medicine, but are known to be associated with poor immune function; examples include TB, herpes, candida and intestinal parasites. However resistance to all infection is reduced in AIDS. Sufferers may succumb to viral, bacterial, fungal, or protozoal infection of any part of the body. They are attacked by many infections at once. At the same time, HIV damage to the brain can cause illness ranging from intense depression to a rapidly progressing dementia.

110

Prognosis

Too little is known about the range of effects caused by HIV to be emphatic about the long-term outcome of infection. Of homosexual men known to be infected, one third have progressed to AIDS within three years. However, people such as haemophiliacs and their wives, whose lifestyles make them less vulnerable, usually remain free of symptoms for very much longer. Many of those known to have encountered HIV show no symptoms of infection, and most of their families also remain well. How long this situation will persist, nobody knows; but it is clear that the disease can be slowed, if not halted, in its progress. It may be that many of those exposed to HIV will remain well indefinitely, but with latency periods already known to last up to nineteen years — effectively, as long as there is evidence of the existence of the virus — it is clearly foolish to make any assertions about the proportion of individuals whose lifespan will be severely curtailed by HIV infection.

What we can assert with confidence is that the prognosis is significantly affected by lifestyle factors. People who have many sexual partners deteriorate relatively more rapidly than those who have one or none; and the disease progresses more rapidly in intravenous drug users (and their babies) than in those who choose a lifestyle which enhances immunity.

Incidence

Any figures on the incidence of AIDS or HIV infection are estimates. Nobody knows how many people are infected. What we do know is that the number of cases is increasing at an exponential rate characteristic of life processes, doubling every ten months in Britain. World-wide, if the current rate of growth were to continue until the end of the century, 32 million will be *known* to be infected with HIV, while the number of people actually infected is likely to be nearer 200 million.

The numbers of cases of AIDS and deaths due to AIDS published by governments are, inevitably, underestimates. It was not until late 1986 that many African governments acknowledged that there was an AIDS problem at all. Diagnosis of AIDS depends on the judgement of individual doctors and their particular definition of the condition. This is influenced by political and social pressures as well as medical knowledge. AIDS is difficult to define in clinical terms because it can produce so many types of illness; in addition, the disease is heavily stigmatized. Because of this, another cause of death may be deliberately selected, or deaths due to HIV infection may be wrongly attributed. If someone dies of a relatively common infection such as a bacterial or viral pneumonia (both of which can develop as a consequence of HIV infection), the underlying AIDS problem may never be observed or recorded. Both of these factors result in underestimation of the size of the problem.

In most countries, there is no legal requirement that forces doctors to report cases of AIDS; it is not a notifiable disease in Britain (although whooping cough, a fairly mild condition, is). So the statistics that are gathered come from voluntary reporting, a notoriously unreliable source of information.

Nevertheless, trends can be identified from the records of clinics which specialize in sexually transmitted disease. In London and in American cities, these clinics report that changes in sexual behaviour appear to have reduced the rate of spread of HIV infection among informed communities. In London, the incidence of gonorrhoea and other sexually transmitted infections has fallen, revealing a general move towards safer sexual practices and reduced numbers of sexual partners.

The apparent reduction in the rate of spread of HIV infection is no cause for complacency, however. A reservoir of infection already exists which is quite sufficient to maintain the epidemic. Because of the delay in emergence of symptoms, many of those infected will not be aware that they could be spreading the disease. The danger of AIDS is here to stay.

Vectors

The vector of HIV is the one most difficult to manage: other people. The virus is transmitted from one person to another in bodily fluids. Attention has been focussed on semen and blood, but HIV has also been found in vaginal secretions, saliva, urine and tears. This means that men can become infected through intercourse with women, deep kissing may transmit the virus, and a wide range of sexual behaviours are now risky.

Any surgical or cosmetic treatment involving penetration of the skin or contamination with another person's fluids, either directly or through faulty hygiene, offers a transmission route for the virus. Transplants offer another route. A few kidney transplant recipients have contracted the disease from the organs they received. One recipient of a temporary skin graft was infected before hasty medical staff learned the result of a routine HIV test on the tissue. Mothers using sperm banks for anonymous donor pregnancies have suffered the same fate. Any transmission of tissue or fluid from another person remains risky until there is a foolproof test for the virus. Such 100 per cent accurate tests are rare in biology.

Public information campaigns have concentrated on some of the sexual means of transmission, advising the use of condoms and spermicidal creams during any act of penetration. While condoms will reduce the risk of infection considerably, they can fail; they are known to fail to protect against pregnancy for about 4 per cent of regular users each year. This figure cannot be translated into a precise estimate for AIDS risk reduction because of the different factors involved in each case, but it clearly reveals that condoms do not offer the prospect of totally safe sex. We believe it is necessary to restrict the transmission of *all* bodily fluids. *Physical contact between strangers is only safe if it is dry.*

Sharing facilities such as baths and pools can bring exposure to traces of other people's body fluids. Well-maintained swimming pools are believed to be safe, but this clearly depends on the precise meaning of 'well-maintained'.

HIV is rapidly killed by chlorine and household bleach, so swimming in a chlorinated pool should not entail risk. Shared jacuzzis should, in our opinion, be avoided; the warm re-circulating water looks too friendly to viruses.

Other potential vectors for HIV include blood-sucking insects. The virus has been found in African bedbugs, although mosquitoes are believed not to present a risk. Whether HIV will spill over into other vectors as it becomes more populous, or whether its nature will change to allow it to use other vectors, is unpredictable. These are possibilities that should not be dismissed.

In the absence of better information, we each have to make up our minds on the degree of risk we are prepared to accept. The problem has not been helped by government officials who make emphatic statements about safety, only to be forced to retract them later as new information emerges. Until we have experienced the full potential of this virus or found a way to master it, it is only sensible to be cautious and err on the side of safety.

With a continually changing virus, we must remain especially vigilant. The Great Plague was difficult to catch when it was *bubonic*, and could be transmitted only by fleas or from direct contact with discharge from buboes (boils in armpits or groin). But when the disease became *pneumonic*, people caught it just by breathing.

113

Positive Action

In the age of AIDS we have to assume that anyone could be carrying the virus, and behave accordingly. Avoidance of the virus is the only certain protection. At present this means avoiding contamination with the bodily fluids or tissues of others from any source which could be suspect. The only people who are safe from sexual transmission are those who are in exclusive, long-term, stable relationships, where neither partner has sex with a third party.

AIDS means that everyone must adapt their behaviour in interpersonal relationships. The social challenge of the virus must be met by developing a social and sexual ethic with more open attitudes and information, but less sexual activity. This is especially relevant for the young; our media banks are contaminated with images of pre-AIDS sexual behaviour that is now dangerous. To promote ignorance or enforced inhibition is no answer; this has always favoured disease. We must be quite clear and unambiguous about what is safe behaviour and what is not.

The principle is simple. Any form of activity that involves mingling body fluids, or contact between any membranes apart from intact skin, is risky. Everyone must face the seriousness of this risk and restrict such activity until they can be completely sure of the safety of their partners.

Young people considering a stable relationship and starting a family need to adopt old-fashioned courtship time-scales, combined with new-fashioned emotional and physical gratification practices. Casual sex and casual pregnancy are out; consenting adults are consenting to much more than ever before. They must focus on what it is they really want from sex. For many it will be the closeness, affection and emotional security that the relationship offers, rather than copulation and orgasms.

Condoms offer the best protection to those who are determined to be sexually active despite the risks. These protect the delicate mucosa at the tip of the penis from viruses secreted by a sexual partner, and protect the man's partner from any viruses he may secrete. (Note the problem of condom failure discussed above.)

Oral sex and kissing also pose problems. Contrary to government assertions, there is evidence that HIV can be transmitted in saliva. Indeed it would be strange if this were not the case, when infectious mononucleosis (glandular fever), another viral disease which attacks white blood cells, is well known to be transmitted in saliva. Other links between the two diseases, including the development of cancers caused by the mononucleosis virus in AIDS sufferers, suggest we should take notice of the association.

However, we must acknowledge the limits of risk. There is no evidence that HIV can be transmitted between different members of the same household, who share cuddles, cutlery and domestic facilities. Nor are you likely to be at risk if your workmate is infected.

The emergence of AIDS among specific high-risk groups led to a false sense of complacency among those who did not identify with these groups. It is important to understand that gays and addicts are not cut off from the rest of society. There is a continuum of contact which embraces us all. Prostitution is a frequent link between the most promiscuous individuals, addicts seeking money to support their habit, and ordinary family men.

While HIV infection is undoubtedly more widespread than is realized, the healthy immune system is capable of mounting some resistance against it. Symptoms are not appearing at the anticipated rate among healthy groups of people who have been exposed to HIV by accident or misfortune rather than lifestyle patterns, notably the wives and children of haemophiliacs infected by contaminated blood products.

We conclude that we are not helpless in the face of this scourge, even when infected by it. Positive action can bring worthwhile results. In addition to specific avoidance measures, you should, of course, live by the tenets of Chapter 2. If you have been exposed to possible infection, warding off other infections by improving your immune function is doubly important.

If you should be unfortunate enough to have the HIV virus, your options are simplified; you must devote your energies to prolonging your life. There is no evidence which proves that any specific course of action has irrefutable benefits, but there is hopeful circumstantial evidence. It has been observed that the course of the syndrome varies widely from one individual to another, and people who decide to maintain a high level of health are able to resist the effects of the virus for much longer than those who do not make this choice.

Beyond individual action, HIV infection must become a notifiable disease. To defeat it, we need accurate knowledge of the ways in which it spreads. To rely on a voluntary system of reporting in combination with a vague definition of the disease could have disastrous consequences.

115

AIDS and Pregnancy

If you know that you are infected with HIV, you should avoid pregnancy. We believe that every woman should have a blood test to check for anti-bodies to HIV as soon as she knows she is pregnant, and if the result is positive she should have an abortion. People infected with the virus should consider sterilization. These proposals may seem draconian, but the tragedy of the birth of babies with AIDS is simply too dreadful to accept. It is likely that every infected mother will transmit the virus to her baby before birth.

Because of the long latency period of HIV it is possible that the effects will not fully emerge until the next generation arrives. This could be a further contribution to the numbers of children who have AIDS in Africa. Infected people who are managing to resist the effects of the virus could produce children who will succumb before they are able to develop their own immune competence.

Not only must infected mothers-to-be face the prospect of giving birth to a baby who will die of multiple infections within a few years, but they also put themselves at additional risk. The immune suppression that occurs during pregnancy accelerates the course of the disease. There can be no sense in hastening one's own death in order to give birth to a child who will shortly die.

Medicine

There is no medical answer to AIDS.

A tremendous research effort is directed towards finding a vaccine. This will prove difficult because the virus changes its antigens so rapidly, and because of the affinity of the virus with the immune system. Any immunological attack on the virus would carry the risk of an auto-immune reaction. A second problem is that it would be extremely difficult to test any vaccine because of the long latency periods involved in HIV infection.

The most hopeful route may lie in attacking the enzyme, reverse transcriptase, which the virus needs to replicate. The success of this strategy will depend upon the precise nature of this enzyme, and how similar it is to enzymes we depend on. Early reports of the effects of AZT, a drug which interferes with the action of reverse transcriptase, suggest that although it can hold up the progression of AIDS, it frequently damages the bone marrow. This is clearly not the sort of drug that could be used to fend off the effects of HIV in the long term.

The prospects for discovery of a drug that will eliminate HIV from the body are slim. No drug has yet been developed that is capable of doing this in any viral infection, let alone one as elusive as HIV.

Some of the resultant opportunistic infections can be treated with antibiotics, and new techniques are increasing secondary treatment success. On the other hand medicines may increase the immune suppression caused by HIV. Some AIDS victims' deaths have been accelerated by inappropriate medical treatment. No treatment can prevent the final immune collapse caused by HIV infection.

Prospects

In the long term the only answer may be to contain the virus in those already infected. If we do this early enough it need not be a traumatic experience, either socially or individually. Obviously it is a tactic which requires discrimination, but this has always been so in outbreaks of plague. It can be an enlightened co-operative action, or one motivated by fear and malice; that is a matter of social choice which should not inhibit consideration of the possibility. Dangerous reaction takes over when the problem can no longer be ignored.

Many primitive attitudes still survive from our past. We may not regard as revolutionary those who propose a natural causation of disease today, but there are religious elements who still encourage the idea of epidemics as 'God's punishment for sinfulness', and it may be that with the failure of medicine and Church, we revert to seeking causes in the malevolence of people. If this is true we will be reacting exactly as we did in 1665 in the wake of the Great Plague. Our answer must be more rational, if only because our enemy has become more persistent and potentially more deadly.

117

10

Herpes

Herpes is the family name for a group of viruses which are transmitted by close body contact (see Chapter 8). Herpes viruses can survive indefinitely in body cells, usually producing no symptoms. They are extremely common; 90 per cent of adults have up to four different kinds of herpes viruses in their bodies.

The virus popularly known as herpes is *Herpes simplex*; it produces sores. *Herpes simplex* Type I tends to affect parts above the waist. Usually, a small area of skin only is affected, most often the margin of one lip (cold sores), but this virus is capable of affecting any part of the body, including the eyes.

Herpes simplex Type II, also known as *Herpes genitalis*, prefers the lower parts of the body, especially the genital area. This is thought to be slightly different form from the virus which produces cold sores on the face, but there is controversy about the degree to which each form can infect other parts of the body. It may be that Type I and Type II are just minor variants on the same theme.

Herpes zoster, another member of the family, causes the familiar childhood disease of chicken-pox. It can recur as shingles when specific immunity has been eroded and general resistance is low. Shingles often develops in transplant recipients and cancer patients taking immunosuppressant drugs.

Epstein-Barr (EB) virus is another member of the herpes family. It produces infectious mononucleosis, also known as glandular fever or 'the kissing disease'. Characteristically, it affects young people who are just becoming sexually active. Epstein-Barr virus attacks the B-cells of the immune system. It can cause a long illness with swollen glands, high fever and depression, but often it produces no discernible symptoms and past infection can only be inferred by the appearance of antibodies to the virus. The crucial factor seems to be the immune status of the person at the time of infection.

Cytomegalovirus (CMV) is less well known, but still common. It causes symptoms similar to glandular fever (EB virus infection) and is often sexually transmitted.

Herpes viruses have the ability to persist in the body for life. They lodge inside cells, their presence undetectable to the immune system while they lie dormant. Then, when the vigilance of the immune system is reduced, they can emerge to multiply and cause symptoms.

Apart from the occasional appearance of sores around the lips when we are exposed to cold winds or under attack by another kind of virus, we are completely unaware of the presence of herpes viruses in our bodies. But if we are unfortunate enough to have *Herpes simplex* in the nerves that serve the genital organs or the eyes, any flare-up can be intensely painful. While it is obviously sensible to try to prevent the virus from entering delicate parts of the body like the genital organs, the most important aspect of dealing with herpes is maintaining a high level of general immunity.

119

Herpex Simplex: Symptoms and Control

Cold sores have been known for thousands of years. They were identified by the Greeks, and the Roman Emperor Tiberius banned kissing in a vain attempt to stop their spread. We can speculate about whether damage by lead poisoning to the immune defences of the Romans caused herpes to be the subject of such imperial attention. Certainly the evidence today suggests that the current herpes epidemic is more a product of disruption to our immune systems than the result of any other type of change.

While cold sores are generally no more than a minor annoyance, herpes lesions on the genital organs or the eyes can be extremely unpleasant. One of the worst aspects of infection is the constant fear of recurrence, which makes sufferers conscious of the problem even when they are free from symptoms. Yet perhaps as many as 50 per cent of people who have one attack of genital herpes never have another. Others have frequent attacks. The difference is entirely in the degree of resistance to the virus that their respective immune systems can muster. When immunity is severely disrupted, as in immunosuppressed people and AIDS sufferers, herpes sores can break out on many parts of the body at once.

Herpes sufferers can often tell when an attack is coming on before there are any signs that anyone else could detect. A localized itchiness or burning sensation can precede the appearance of the small reddened bumps that turn into the characteristic cluster of herpes blisters. After about forty-eight hours, these blisters rupture to form weeping open sores. Within a week or perhaps two, they begin to heal and gradually disappear.

A severe attack will be accompanied by the other familiar signs of virus infection – fever, malaise, headache, depression. These show that the body is going through its normal anti-virus routine: producing interferons, raising the temperature, manufacturing antibodies. This will not completely vanquish the virus, which can make itself undetectable by hiding in cells, but it will shorten the acute phase of the illness. It will also ensure that each attack is likely to be less severe than the first. Unless it is severely damaged, the immune system eventually wins; herpes stops recurring after an unpredictable length of time.

Open herpes sores shed large quantities of virus, but the discomfort they cause tends to deter people from having sexual contact while they are suffering from active symptoms. At other times, herpes is not readily transmitted; herpes sufferers can live for years with partners who do not have attacks. It is often not clear how a particular individual came to develop herpes, although sexual transmission of genital herpes does undoubtedly occur.

Contact with herpes sores on any part of the body can transmit infection. It is possible to spread infection from one part of one's own body to another by touching the sores and transferring virus particles on the fingers. In some cases, sharing a towel with a sufferer is sufficient to cause infection. Virus particles can be transmitted via wrestling mats and probably even lavatory seats. But, as with all infections, whether you begin to suffer symptoms will depend on your ability to resist the virus; and whether you suffer recurring attacks depends on the effectiveness of your immune system.

Herpes and Sex

Diseases that can develop spontaneously and cause pain in the sexual organs are often linked with sexual problems. Anxiety about sex could trigger your herpes, and herpes often causes anxiety about sex. This is a difficult problem to resolve. The most difficult aspect of it, for most people, is to achieve the honesty and trust required to cope with herpes in a new sexual relationship. Some avoid the problem by remaining celibate; perhaps for them, this was the desired end, achieved by a regrettably painful means. So do not be surprised if you develop a persistent outbreak of herpes after the breakup of an important sexual relationship. As your emotional wounds heal, your herpes will also come under control.

Sexual behaviour and contraceptive practice are both involved in the rise of *Herpes genitalis*; but it is to be hoped that the new AIDS-inspired awareness of the importance of effective protection against sexually transmitted disease will inhibit the spread of herpes.

121

Positive Action

Many herpes sufferers point to stress as the most important trigger which leads to attacks. Exhaustion from pressures at work or at home, emotional upheavals and depression are often linked with the appearance or re-emergence of symptoms. Many women find that outbreaks are more frequent around the menstrual period. So stress management, and the need to recognize and reject unacceptably stressful situations, are clearly important to those at risk of herpes flare-ups. Of course it is also important to maintain a high level of immunity by following the advice given in Chapter 2.

Drugs and Medicine

There are no drugs that can cure herpes, but acyclovir (Zovirax) can often reduce the intensity and duration of the symptoms. It is available on prescription and should be used as symptoms begin. Drugs which reduce inflammation could make your herpes worse, so do not use anything other than specific anti-viral creams.

The use of oral contraceptives may contribute to the genital herpes epidemic in a number of ways, making the membranes more vulnerable to infection and probably reducing general immunity to viral infection. Herpes sufferers should therefore change to an alternative contraceptive method.

Limiting the Spread of Herpes

People with outbreaks of herpes sores on *any* parts of their bodies are likely to be infectious. The liquid that weeps from the sores is rich in viruses which will try to invade other flesh. It is irresponsible, therefore, to have any form of intimate physical contact with another person if you have active herpes, unless you live with that person and your problem is shared. Never allow the sores or the fluid secreted from them to come into contact with any part of another person's body, or even another part of your own body.

If your partner, a friend, or a member of your family has active herpes, avoid using towels or clothing that may have come into contact with the lesions. If you have active herpes, keep your towel and clothing strictly segregated from everyone else's.

122

The *Herpes genitalis* Epidemic – Why is it Spreading Now?

A curious feature of the herpes problem is that the familiar cold sore, Type I herpes, seems to be less common, at least among children. In 1953, 85 per cent of school-age children had antibodies to herpes in their blood; twelve years later, this figure had fallen to 41 per cent. We can only speculate about the reason for this: possibly it is the result of increasing affluence, preventing the occurrence of cold sores in the families which had 'never had it so good'. However, it could be a result of changing play patterns among children which limit the spread of all forms of herpes virus, because other members of the herpes family are also less often transmitted between children than they were some decades ago.

It could be that increased vulnerability to genital herpes (estimated to be rising at the rate of 12 per cent per annum in Britain) is related to decreased immunity to Type I herpes. As with chicken-pox, it may be better to suffer trivial infection in childhood and be free from more severe outbreaks in adulthood.

11

Allergies and Auto-immunity

Allergies and auto-immune diseases are more common today than ever before and the incidence of these problems is increasing steadily. The basic cause of both types of illness is a failure of immune discrimination. This breakdown results from exposure to increasing quantities and numbers of different novel substances which pollute every part of our environment.

Allergy is an excessive or inappropriate reaction to a normally harmless substance. For example, when the immune system responds to pollen grains as though they were dangerous pathogens, the result is hay fever; when it treats particular types of food, or the chemicals they contain, as though they were poisons, the result is food intolerance. Allergies can develop to virtually any substance, natural or synthetic, which enters the body by any means. The substances which trigger allergies are known as allergens.

Respiratory allergic reactions are usually, but not always, triggered by airborne allergens. These include hay fever, asthma, and perennial rhinitis (chronic runny nose). Chronic sinus or lung problems may be allergic in origin. Allergic ear problems include secretory otitis media, which causes earache, blocked ears and hearing loss.

Conjunctivitis – sore, itchy, swollen, or red eyes – may develop as part of a pattern of respiratory allergy, as in hay fever, or as an independent allergic reaction.

Allergic skin reactions include eczema, urticaria (nettle rash or hives), and dermatitis. These rashes may be itchy or sore, sometimes covering large areas of the body. Angioedoema is an allergic reaction in deeper layers of the skin which produces swelling and sometimes pain, often in the lips.

Food allergies can produce a very wide range of symptoms from bloating and abdominal pain to behaviour problems. Food allergy has been blamed for much sub-clinical malaise, a feeling of general, pervasive unwellness, and for widespread emotional disturbance.

Auto-immune conditions result from inappropriate reactions to internal stimuli. Whereas in allergic conditions there is an excessive reaction to external stimuli, in auto-immunity the body attacks components within itself – self-antigens to which reactions should be suppressed. Conditions which result include rheumatoid arthritis, ulcerative colitis, juvenile-onset diabetes, multiple sclerosis, some types of anaemia, Myasthenia gravis, systemic lupus erythematosus (SLE) and many more.

Sometimes there are clear links between allergy and auto-immunity. Auto-immune symptoms can develop when sufferers are exposed to substances, particularly drugs and foods to which they are sensitive, and cease when these substances are removed. In other cases there may be no clear link; an auto-immune process may seem to begin spontaneously, though usually there are links with severe stress, virus infection, or metabolic change.

Common Allergens

Allergic disorders can usually be linked to particular triggers (allergens) which set off the illness. The most common allergens are listed below, with the types of reaction they are most likely to trigger.

House-dust mites: These microscopic creatures live on skin scales, shed constantly from our bodies. They accumulate in our homes, especially in beds. Mites or debris from them are particularly linked with asthma, perennial rhinitis (chronic runny nose), chronic conjunctivitis (red eye), and the exacerbation of seasonal allergies such as hay fever.

Pollens: These produce symptoms from late February to August, peaking in June and July. Grass pollens cause the most frequent problems, hence the name for the common allergic disorder, hay fever. The combination of sneezing, runny eyes, sore throat, and streaming nose can be difficult to distinguish from a cold unless it persists for a long period or recurs at the same time every year. Tree and wild-flower pollens also produce these symptoms in some people. The pattern of species causing allergic reactions varies between individuals.

Mildews: Spores from mildews can trigger a range of allergic reactions, notably asthma. The problem is particularly severe in late summer (July to September). The mildews involved may live on any plant matter (e.g. in grain fields and stores), in buildings, damp wood and plaster, old books, or other organic substances.

Animal danders: These include products, particularly hair and minute fragments of skin, from cats, dogs, horses, or other animals. The most common reaction is asthma.

Other airborne substances: This group includes chemicals such as pesticides (particularly linked with asthma), household products such as washing powder and sprays, and many chemicals used in industry. While asthma is the best-documented reaction, members of this group may set off a wide range of allergic reactions. They also make a significant contribution to the development of allergic reactions to other substances.

125

Foods: Allergy can be triggered by a huge range of foods, particularly dairy produce and eggs. Foods have been linked with all types of allergic reaction in sensitive people, including asthma, eczema, rheumatoid arthritis and other joint disorders, vomiting and indigestion, and emotional and mental problems such as depression and even schizophrenia.

Food additives/pollutants: Colours, preservatives, and flavour enhancers are relatively frequent allergy triggers. Reactions vary from inflammation and swelling of the lips and mouth, through hyperactivity and delinquency, to asthma. There is little systematic information on the role played by process, storage and pesticide residues in triggering allergies.

Drugs/medicines: Drugs can trigger a wide range of allergic reactions. When given by injection, some drugs can cause anaphylactic shock, a rapid and sometimes fatal allergic reaction involving severe asthma. Penicillin and products given for densensitization to allergens are the most common culprits. Many types of medicine can set off allergies in sensitive individuals. Aspirin is a fairly common trigger. Even natural products such as insulin are capable of setting off allergic reactions. Skin reactions such as urticaria are particularly common, but asthma and other allergic diseases are not unusual. Serious auto-immune disease is a well-recognized adverse effect of medication.

Chemicals and metals: The type of allergic reaction induced by chemicals depends largely on the way they enter the body. Contact determatitis, an allergic skin rash at the point of contact, is particularly common, but sneezing and more severe allergic reactions can occur with inhaled chemicals. The range of substances capable of inducing allergic reactions is tremendous, but some of the more common culprits are nickel, enzymes (in detergents) and pesticides.

Insect bites and stings: Bee stings, in particular, can provoke violent allergic reactions in sensitive people. The first sting may produce nothing more than discomfort, but subsequent stings may precipitate a sudden and severe illness. Anaphylaxis resulting from a sting causes extreme asthma with swelling of the throat and a precipitous drop in blood pressure. Emergency treatment with adrenalin is essential. Because of the seriousness of this situation, people who are allergic to bee stings should ask their doctors for desensitization treatment.

Susceptibility to Allergy and Auto-immunity

Genetic Predisposition

Suffers from allergic and auto-immune conditions usually have a higher than normal proportion of sufferers among their close relatives. Particular genetic markers have been identified which seem to predispose some individuals to these types of illness, though how they operate is not known. But genetic predispositions are translated into individual characteristics only when suitable environmental conditions exist. Vulnerability to allergic illness means that the person is more likely to develop symptoms *when exposed to the environmental pressures that tend to induce it.*

As the environmental conditions which induce allergic reactions become more widespread, more of those who are genetically prone to allergy or auto-immune breakdown will succumb. This is precisely what is happening at the moment. With mounting pressure on immune memory systems, less sensitive people start to suffer from allergies. Everyone is at risk; our genes merely determine the degree of risk posed for each one of us.

Early Experience

For some decades, it has been observed that bottle-fed babies are especially likely to suffer from allergic problems, notably eczema. Mother's milk contains immunoglobulins which strengthen the baby's immune system and tend to prevent the development of allergies, while cow's milk is a common allergen which is particularly likely to cause problems when the immune system is immature. Some of the most recent studies, however, reveal a reversal of the accepted pattern. Babies who are breast-fed for six months or more are now showing *increased* allergy problems. Eczema and, to a lesser degree, hay fever, are increased by long periods of breast-feeding.

The explanation for this disturbing finding must lie in the nature of the breast milk. In many parts of Britain, the average mother's milk contains such high levels of pesticides and other dangerous chemicals that a baby would receive more than the maximum daily dose permitted by the World Health Organization. Under such circumstances, the development of allergic reactions is only to be expected.

Eczema in infancy is often a sign of other allergic problems to come in later life. If immune discrimination begins to fail early, recovery can be difficult.

Early Medical Treatment

Anaesthetics given in the first two years of life have been found to predispose to the later development of respiratory allergies, probably because administration of a general anaesthetic damages the membranes that line the respiratory tract.

Infection

Virus infections seem to increase susceptibility to many allergic and auto-immune reactions. Auto-immune disease affecting the joints, kidneys, pancreas or other organs can follow virus infection. Infection of the gut by the fungus, candida (thrush), has been linked with the development of food allergies.

Many separate mechanisms could account for these links. Infection of membranes damages mast cells, leading to loss of discrimination and a partial failure of their gate-keeping function. This allows allergens to penetrate into the bloodstream, where antibodies will be formed against them, which will change the mast cells' responses when they later encounter the same allergen. In addition, acute infection would alter the functional balance of the immune system as a whole, tending to increase the activities of T-helper lymphocytes and reduce T-suppressor activity. This would reduce tolerance to antigens within the system in a general way. Finally, immune complexes, or antigen–antibody combinations formed by immune-system reactions to infections, can lodge in parts of the body including the kidney and joints and induce inflammation and damage. The reasons for this reaction are not known, but the relative proportions of antigen to antibody within the body seem to be crucial. This also suggests that the balance of helper to suppressor lymphocyte function is disturbed in auto-immune disease. The implication is that people who suffer from allergic or auto-immune conditions will benefit from action which increases their resistance to infection.

128

Incidence

The prevalence of allergic disorders has increased greatly in recent years. The table below shows the rise in consultations with general practitioners for allergic problems between 1955–6 and 1981–2. (Figures are for consultations per 1,000 patients per year, from *Morbidity Statistics from General Practice, 1981–2.*)

The most marked increases in allergic illness are among children. In one long-term study of two generations, eczema rates were 2.2 per 1,000 in people born in 1946, rising to 12.3 per 1,000 in their first-born offspring. Similarly, asthma rates among children under four years of age rose from 6.2 per 1,000 to 18.9 per 1,000. The death-rate due to asthma is rising despite increasingly sophisticated and effective treatment, yet at the turn of the century doctors maintained that asthma did not kill.

Of the auto-immune conditions, the rise in juvenile-onset diabetes is the best documented. In 1956, 0.2 per 1,000 eleven-year-old children were dependent on insulin injections. The corresponding rate twelve years later was 0.6 per 1,000, and twenty-five years later it had risen to 1.3 per

Condition	1955	1971	1981
Dermatitis and eczema	24.3	42.8	45.6
Asthma	(no data)	9.6	17.8
Hay fever	(no data)	11.0	19.7
Conjunctivitis (age 0–4) (age 5–14)	19.2	68.6 18.9	116.5 33.0

1,000 in children of the same age. This represents a very serious increase in auto-immune disease, because diabetes markedly reduces life-expectancy, and is very detrimental to the quality of life both for diabetics and for those who live with them. While asthma and diabetes are more common today than ever before, they have been known for thousands of years. Some other allergic disorders are products of recent cultural changes.

The industrial revolution and the expansion of the chemical industry which followed it has had many undesirable effects on health, one of which is the development of hay fever. The first documented cases of hay fever were observed in the early years of the nineteenth century; before this, there is no record of such a condition. Even in the late nineteenth century, hay fever was a rare occurrence, and in much of Europe it was not believed to exist at all.

Allergies in general are more common in urban areas than in the country, although exposure to chemicals used on farm land can precipitate the development of lasting allergic problems. Few people develop allergies in unpolluted regions such as mountains and the seaside, unless they are frequently exposed to mouldy hay or other sources of potent allergens.

Food allergies can occur at any age, though they have been most closely studied in hyperactive children. This is a controversial area because many members of the medical profession, influenced by the food industry through front organizations such as the British Nutrition Foundation, express the view that allergy to food and chemicals in food is very rare indeed, while independent clinical ecologists argue that it is much more common than generally recognized. Problems of measurement and definition complicate the issue. Generally poor nutrition and the substitution of chemicals for real

129

food, adds to the difficulty of deciding what the basis of an apparently diet-related problem might be.

Positive Action

Reducing Susceptibility

The Norwegian health ministry's analogy for allergic illness provides a useful starting-point for understanding what has to be done to reduce it. They produced the image of a bucket which represents our capacity to cope with substances we encounter. Every potential allergen, every chemical, every new molecule that enters our body helps to fill the bucket. Each person's bucket has an individual capacity, and some substances will have a disproportionate bucket-filling effect in relation to the quantities that enter the body. When the bucket overflows, we experience allergic symptoms.

The most effective action we can take to reduce the severity of allergy problems is to start emptying the bucket. This means that we have to reduce our exposure to *all* potential allergens in order to reduce the reaction to any particular one.

The size of the bucket is not constant; it changes with changes in lifestyle. Poor nutrition and other aspects of lifestyle that interfere with efficient immune function will tend to shrink the bucket. Emotional stress will make it more liable to spill. The general advice on lifestyle given in Chapter 2 is important to all allergy sufferers because adopting these patterns of behaviour will increase resistance to allergy by effectively enlarging the bucket.

However, while the principles of action against specific allergies are quite straightforward, in practice there is no simple answer to the solution of such problems. For example, it may do little good to try to reduce the body's reaction to one particular substance such as grass pollen. Although this will limit the symptoms of grass-pollen allergy when the bucket is being filled very fast with this particular allergen, other allergic problems are likely to develop if the bucket stays on the verge of spilling.

The bucket model also implies that is possible to become effectively tolerant of allergens even when they are present in large quantities in the environment, thereby reducing their effects. This is obviously valuable to people such as hay-fever sufferers who cannot hope to avoid the allergen to which they react. Since any substance which regularly causes allergic symptoms is likely to fill the bucket particularly fast, it does make sense to identify and avoid these triggers whenever possible.

Specific Action to Reduce Allergy

House-dust Mite

This is the most common respiratory allergen throughout the world, affecting humans wherever they settle, wear clothes and build permanent homes. Whether your problem is asthma, hay fever, a perpetually runny nose or blocked-up head, you may be reacting to house-dust mites.

The highest numbers of mites are found in the bedroom, in bedding, mattresses, pillows, soft toys, on the floor, in the dust on the dressing-table and skirting boards. Lying in bed, we are exposed to high concentrations of them.

To reduce the level of dust mite, all surfaces need to be kept very clean and free from dust. Ideally, allergy sufferers should have Norwegian-style bedrooms, with varnished or painted wood and rugs which can be washed regularly rather than thick-pile fitted carpets.

The bed is particularly important, containing, on average, about 10,000 mites. Bedding made from synthetic fibre is less attractive to the mite, and it can be washed frequently (but not with biological detergents because they are often linked with allergy; a safe washing powder is Ecover, available from wholefood shops). Bedding or pillows containing feathers or down should be avoided. Pillows should also be washed. The mattress should be covered completely with a plastic sheet so that a mite population does not build up in it. Foam mattresses are less attractive to mites than interior spring types.

Vacuum cleaning is very helpful but the allergy sufferer should try to get someone else to do it. Clean thoroughly and frequently around and under the bed and vacuum the mattress when changing the sheets. Always get someone else to empty the vacuum cleaner. Use a damp mop or cloth to keep all surfaces free of dust. Mites thrive in warm, dark, damp conditions. Keeping the bedroom well aired, hanging bedding in the sun, and avoiding gas or paraffin heaters that produce water vapour will help keep their numbers down.

131

Activity

While the general advice in Chapter 2 is appropriate for most allergy sufferers, vigorous activity can precipitate asthma attacks. However, while it is essential to take precautions against triggering asthma, the correct type of exercise will prove beneficial. The key is moderation: always stop short of precipitating an attack. But the more you do at this level, the more you will be able to do, and the more your health will benefit.

In general, short periods of one to two minutes' rapid activity followed by rest are most suitable for asthmatics, not continuous strenuous activity like running. Stop–start games like badminton can be fine, while activities such as cycling, where you can alternate between effort and rest, are also good. However, protection from cold air is essential; no asthmatic should exercise outside in cold weather. Swimming and walking will be beneficial, and should not cause problems unless the sufferer gets cold. Combine brisk walking with deep breathing from the abdomen in unpolluted air for maximum benefit.

132

Diet

The organic wholefood diet described in Chapter 2 is particularly important for allergy sufferers. It is not infrequently found that while a commercial product is linked with symptoms, its pure equivalent is harmless. If you believe that you suffer from multiple food allergies, or you have failed to find the trigger for your allergic reactions, adopting a pure and nutritionally adequate diet could solve the problem.

This type of diet is free from all the additives that have been specifically linked with allergic problems. Anyone who is susceptible to allergies would be wise to avoid as many food additives and chemicals as possible. A few are believed to be completely harmless and these include, for example, E160 and E161, which are naturally occurring plant colours related to vitamin A, often added to margarine.

Sensitivity to particular foods or food components should not, however, be dismissed. Gluten in grains and lactose in milk, for example (whether or not they are pure), can induce allergic reactions in sensitive people. The only way to check these possibilities if you have reason to believe that your problems are associated with them is to give up entirely eating suspect foods for a minimum of a week, while keeping a diary of your symptoms. If the symptoms disappear within a few days of giving up the food, and return with redoubled force the first time you eat it again, then your suspicions will be confirmed and you would be wise to eat that food only in small quantities, and only occasionally.

The problem with food allergy is that it is all too easy to suspect falsely a wide range of foods and end up eating a limited and nutritionally inadequate diet, which will then exacerbate allergy problems. This danger must not be underestimated. Food allergy sufferers should also beware of classifying all foods of a particular type as hazardous because they have experienced problems with some of them. For example, sensitivity to peanuts does not imply sensitivity to almonds and other nuts. It is essential to test very carefully to identify precisely what causes problems, not to guess or make assumptions.

Whatever the specific allergic or auto-immune problem we confront, we should not forget the underlying cause. Disruption of the ecological balance within the outside environment as well as our internal environment damages the immune system. This issue is the subject of the last section of this book; it is one that most clinicians ignore. The rising prevalence of allergies and the failure of medicine to prevent the misery they cause is just part of the cost we pay for a way of life that does not meet our real needs.

12

Reducing
Cancer Risks

Causes

Cancers occur when the cells in any part of the body begin to reproduce at an excessive rate. Such cells are themselves abnormal and may be detected and destroyed by a healthy immune system. However, when their numbers grow too large, they become capable of suppressing immune reactions, so the most important task facing the immune system is to prevent them from proliferating in the first place.

The abnormal growth patterns characteristic of different cancers are directed by genetic material within the cells, which does not operate as it should. Sometimes, it seems that genes which are normally dormant (oncogenes) are switched on. When they take over the direction of the cell, they create cancers. Oncogenes may be activated by damage to the genetic material in the nucleus of the cell.

Damage to a cell's genetic material can have many causes. The most common culprit is the action of cancer-generating chemicals, or carcinogens. There are many thousands of known carcinogens, and undoubtedly much greater numbers of substances which are unrecognized carcinogens. They are present in small quantities in virtually every part of our environment. The best-known and single most important source of carcinogens today is tobacco, but others range from the rare toxic metal, beryllium, to chemicals used in the production of plastics.

The effects of many carcinogens take decades to emerge, a feature which makes recognition very difficult. To add to the problem, there are interactions between carcinogens; some cancers require the action of an *initiator*, which makes the cell vulnerable, and a *promoter*, which actually sets off the cancer process. In our chemically polluted environment, there can be little hope of identifying all the initiator/promoter pairs to which we may be exposed, especially as testing for carcinogens rarely includes pairs or groups of chemicals.

Radiation – whether from the nuclear industry, nuclear weapons or medical X-rays – can induce cancers by direct bombardment of the genetic material of the cell with sub-atomic particles. This can cause breaks and other abnormalities in the crucial molecular parts of the genetic instruction sequences which direct the development of the cell. The bone marrow seems especially vulnerable to radiation, so leukaemia and rarer types of bone-marrow cancer such as myeloma are particularly likely to result from this type of damage.

135

Some viruses can also induce cancerous changes in the cells they infect. One is the wart virus, which has been linked with cervical cancer. Others are carcinogenic only when the immune system is failing, as in AIDS.

Carcinogens may induce specific cancers such as the type of mesothelioma associated with asbestos, or they may increase vulnerability to one or many relatively common cancers, as in the case of cigarette smoke. If the effect is to increase the numbers of cancers which are already common, it can be very difficult to demonstrate any link, and the hazards of important carcinogens may not be recognized. Links between breast cancer and oral contraceptives are particularly difficult to prove because breast cancer is so common that a proportionately small rise in incidence may not be detected even if that small proportion represents many deaths.

It is often impossible to establish the cause of any individual's cancer. It might be due to childhood play on a beach near a nuclear reprocessing plant, or to some aspect of diet or lifestyle, or any other potential cause. General trends can be established by looking at different cancer rates in different populations. These reveal the operation of environmental or cultural/lifestyle factors, though they may not accurately pinpoint the ones that are important. For example, much valuable information has been gathered from studies of Chinese people living in Hawaii and other parts of the USA (in progressively more Americanized groups). Usually, it is necessary to look at the pattern of evidence from many different sources before a cause for cancer can be established.

Nevertheless, statistical studies show that about 80 per cent of the cancers we suffer are potentially avoidable. In theory, we could reduce our rate of each type of cancer to that experienced by the group or country that has the *lowest* risk by adopting the aspects of lifestyle that protect those people, and avoiding those things that make higher risk groups vulnerable. Even if we were not able to reduce our overall cancer rate to one fifth of what it is now, just changing our lifestyles in the appropriate ways would cut the suffering and mortality due to cancer very dramatically. As a bonus, we would also suffer less illness of other types, because – predictably – the positive health rules that have come out of research into cancer are very similar to those derived from research into heart disease and many other avoidable ills from which we suffer excessively. The avoidance of potential carcinogens is part of the answer to the cancer problem. The second, equally important, part is maintaining our defences against cancer at the highest possible level.

Among the body's defences are genetic repair systems operating at the cellular level, detoxifying systems which scavenge potentially carcinogenic substances from the body and the constantly vigilant killer cells of the immune system which patrol the body, picking off abnormal cells as they discover them. The efficiency of these protective systems depends largely on the factors discussed in Chapter 2.

Symptoms

During the period when a cancer is just starting to develop and lifestyle action is most beneficial, there are not likely to be any symptoms. In any case, it is rarely possible for a lay person to recognize the signs of development of a cancer. How it might eventually reveal its presence will vary according to the site and type of cancer. Some are quite localized, others disseminated; some form palpable growths on or in normal organs, others are apparent only from changes in the nature or function of a particular body tissue. Eventually, most cancers spread, forming offshoots (metastases) in different parts of the body.

The one sign that is common to all serious cancers is a progressive loss of health; why this happens is not usually known. There is often immune suppression which occurs independently of any drug therapy, and this increases vulnerability to infections. Cancer patients usually suffer substantial weight loss when the disease is well established. Again, the reason for this is often unknown.

Incidence

Cancer is the second most important cause of death in Britain and most of the developed world, accounting for about 20 per cent of mortality. The number of deaths registered as due to cancer is likely to be an underestimate, since fatal illness can result from drastic attempts to deal with cancers, and the immune suppression resulting both from the cancer and its treatment will raise the risk of death from infection. Thus cancer may cause death directly or indirectly, but only in the former case is cancer likely to be recorded as the cause of death.

In England and Wales, the most frequently fatal cancers are those of the lung and windpipe, accounting for 26,000 deaths per year among men and 10,000 among women. The overwhelming majority of these are, or were, cigarette smokers. Next in the mortality hierarchy for women comes breast cancer. This kills about 13,500 each year. Cancers of the rectum and colon come next, with 8,000 male and 9,000 female deaths each year. Prostate cancer, affecting only men, accounts for over 6,000 deaths per year. Stomach cancer accounts for 6,000 male deaths, 4,000 among women. Immune-system cancers kill about 9,000 people per year, just slightly more men than women. Leukaemia, one of this group, is the only type of cancer which is relatively common among children.

Between them, the types listed above account for around 70 per cent of all British cancer deaths. These cancers have been linked with a range of different aspects of lifestyle and life experience.

Positive Action

To the degree that our protective systems cover the whole of our bodies, a general, across-the-board reduction of cancer risk can be achieved by enhancing the efficiency of these systems. The principles are explained in Chapter 2, but research into cancer has highlighted some particular features. If your

137

personal, medical, or family history leads you to suspect that you could be at particular risk of developing cancer, concentrating on the aspects of lifestyle noted below will reduce the risk further.

Tobacco

The links between cancer and cigarette smoking may seem too well known to be worth repeating. No rational person who is concerned to avoid cancer would smoke cigarettes. What is less well known is that 30 per cent of *all* cancers may be attributed to smoking. The risk is not just to the lungs and respiratory system, but to the pancreas, cervix, liver and other organs.

Smoking acts in tandem with other factors to produce cancers. Cancers of the liver and digestive tract are increased in people who drink and smoke. Smoking increases the risk of cancer in people exposed to asbestos or radiation. It increases vulnerability to the carcinogenic effects of polluted city air. And it makes the body less able to absorb nutrients that can protect from cancer.

As we have already noted, tobacco in other forms is also carcinogenic. Pipe smoking is associated with cancer of the lip. Chewing tobacco causes cancers of the mouth, lip and throat. Snuff causes cancers of the nose and sinuses. There is no way you can use tobacco and not face an increased risk of cancer.

Diet

According to Dr John Berg of the Cancer Epidemiology Centre, Iowa, 'Any dietary imbalance, especially one affecting metabolically active tissue, may increase the risk of cancer.' It is especially important that the diet should include sufficient vitamins A, C and E and folic acid; and the minerals selenium and zinc.

A highly processed Western diet is deficient in many nutrients. It is significant that Scotland, with a very unbalanced diet and the lowest recorded consumption of fresh vegetables per head in the world, has a spectacularly high cancer rate. Indeed, in Britain generally, tobacco smoke and other carcinogens with known and measured effects are many times more likely to produce cancers than in countries such as France, where the national diet is more varied and includes far more fresh vegetables.

There are many converging lines of evidence that pinpoint fresh green, yellow or red vegetables as valuable protectors against cancer. They will be especially effective if they are organically produced, for this enhances the trace mineral content. If you produce your own vegetables, ensure that potential deficiencies of such elements as selenium and iodine are remedied by the use of organic seaweed fertilizers.

Seafoods and seaweed (including kelp tablets) are particularly beneficial because they provide nutrients that may not be readily available from other sources. The Japanese, who traditionally eat large quantities of seaweed and other seafoods, have the lowest recorded rates of many kinds of cancer, and very low rates of the cancers which are common in Britain. For example, Japan has a breast cancer death-rate (age-adjusted) that is one fifth of Britain's, and colon cancer rates which are similarly low. However, over recent decades, the Japanese diet has been changing, becoming more like ours, and breast and colon cancers have begun to rise.

Certain micronutrients have been shown to influence susceptibility to specific cancers, while others affect overall cancer rates. The relationships identified below have emerged from epidemiological and clinical research; we can expect that more links with micronutrients will be discovered as scientists continue to study the statistics. Cancer is generally associated with long-term low-level micronutrient imbalances which impair the body's protective system.

Selenium deficiency predisposes to all types of cancer, presumably because selenium plays an essential role in detoxification systems. Long-term low-level zinc deficiency probably increases the risk of all cancers. It has been specifically linked with prostate and oesophageal cancers. Iodine deficiency makes women more vulnerable to breast cancer. There is an association between goitre, a well-known sign of iodine deficiency, and breast cancer. Molybdenum, a trace element which is essential to human metabolism and often lost in food processing, seems to protect against oesophageal cancers.

If you eat plenty of the foods recommended in Chapter 2, your diet will provide these important trace micronutrients.

The other side of the diet coin is the avoidance of potential dietary carcinogens and of eating patterns that increase the risk of cancer. Particularly strong associations have been found between eating habits and cancers of the breast, colon and rectum. These are linked with diets rich in meat, dairy produce, saturated (hard) fats and sugar. Such diets also tend to be deficient in unrefined carbohydrate. In other words, these are cancers that result from a typical refined Western diet.

The correlations between the incidence of breast cancer, the incidence of colon cancer and meat consumption in different countries are very strong indeed at 0.84 (the maximum correlation – a perfect match – is 1.0). The implication is that modern meat (particularly beef) contains substances that can be carcinogenic. We suggest that these carcinogens probably come from substances that the animal was exposed to during its lifetime, and which were concentrated in its body, mainly in fat and the internal organs. Toxins also accumulate in animal products such as milk; if animals' everyday feed contains a little of some carcinogen, their bodies and milk will come to contain a much higher concentration of it.

Processed food adds to the problem. It passes slowly through the gut, so any carcinogens linger in close contact with the walls of the colon. Cells subjected to this sort of treatment over decades get damaged. In addition, on a processed diet the gut is short of protective substances, ranging from micronutrients to the types of fibre that are essential to maintain a healthy gut.

The situation is more complicated with breast cancer. The concentration of varied carcinogens derived from animal products in the woman's milk ducts could explain the observed dietary link. Mammary tumours are common and becoming more frequent in many species of animals in human care, but they are much rarer in wild animals which are not exposed to carcinogens produced by human industry.

Cancer of the breast is more common in fatter women, and it is associated with high levels of female sex hormones, particularly oestradiol. The cyclic changes in these hormones produce corresponding changes in the breast which could cause deposition of fat-soluble carcinogens in the milk ducts. On average, women who eat high-fat, high-sugar and high-meat diets are substantially fatter than those who choose wholefood, vegetarian and other prudent diets. Meat-eaters produce more oestrogens than vegetarians, and so are at higher risk. But frequent consumption of fried potatoes, sweet puddings and white bread and butter has been found to be particularly hazardous for vegetarian women prone to breast cancer.

Pollutants in Food

Our food contains many potential carcinogens and substances that could undermine our immune defences. There are also incalculable possibilities for interaction between these substances, making them more potent collectively than they would be when assessed separately. The Western diet and environment includes an enormous range of chemicals whose effects are unknown.

A few food chemicals have been proved carcinogenic to the satisfaction of most of the scientific community. In some cases, these chemicals are still to be found as additives or contaminants in foods. Saccharin is one example; its association with bladder cancer in animals has been recognized for many decades; and while the evidence on human carcinogenicity is not conclusive, this may reflect the shortcomings of research methods more than the safety of the chemical.

Carcinogens in food can take a variety of forms, often produced in processing. Contamination of polished rice with the talc and asbestos used in polishing leads to a special risk of stomach and intestinal tumours in people who eat a lot of white rice. This is yet another reason for eating nutritionally superior and better tasting natural brown rice. The polycyclic hydrocarbons produced by smoking fish and grilling beef are suspected to be the cause of excess stomach cancers in heavy consumers of smoked fish, and of bowel cancers in frequent steak-eaters. Heavily salted foods, dried fish, and traditional pickles eaten in Scandinavia, China and Japan have been linked with oesophageal and stomach cancers. The most dangerous carcinogenic food contaminant is probably aflatoxin, which causes liver cancer in many tropical areas. Fortunately, in Britain we are spared this particular threat.

Diet is undoubtedly a major contributor to cancer risks, but it is a risk factor that can very easily be eliminated. If we simply replace a significant proportion of the meat and dairy produce in our everyday diet with fresh fish and organic vegetables (preferably eaten raw), our vulnerability to many cancers would be much reduced.

Weight

Excessive quantities of body fat are linked with increased rates of cancers. Fat stores produce oestrogen in women, so it is to be expected that oestrogen-linked cancers – endometrial, ovarian and breast cancers – would also be linked with obesity. Gall-bladder cancer is also more common in overweight people. Many man-made toxins and pollutants are soluble in fat, which acts as a store in the body for substances that cannot be safely metabolized. Chronic exposure to such substances would increase cancer risks; thus both weight gain and cancer could result from problems caused by pollution.

141

Adopting the lifestyle advice given in Chapter 2 and the dietary suggestions above will ensure that excess weight will gradually diminish and disappear. Going on 'slimming' diets will do more harm than good. If you are overweight, the simple answer is to adopt a healthy eating pattern with plenty of fresh natural food, avoiding all sugar and other sweeteners (irrespective of the number of calories they contain), and gradually to increase your activity level. This type of strategy will lead to a permanent loss of superfluous fat.

Drink

Pollution of the water supply can increase cancer risks. Lead, a common contaminant of soft-water supplies in older city houses, is associated with cancers of the stomach, intestines, ovary, kidney and immune system. It makes sense to replace lead plumbing wherever you find it and, until this is done, to remove metals from your water with a purifier.

Alcohol is not likely to cause problems if it is used in moderation. However, alcohol interacts with other carcinogens, both by interfering with liver function and increasing the penetration of carcinogens into the membranes of the mouth and throat. For example, if you smoke and drink your risks of cancer are substantially higher than if you only drink. Excessive drinking causes cancer of the liver – along with other types of liver damage, particularly cirrhosis. The type of alcoholic beverage is of some slight relevance; vodka is apparently less carcinogenic than most whiskies.

Alcohol is used in other forms besides beverages and these, too, have been linked with cancer. Strongly alcoholic mouthwashes, in particular, have been observed to cause cancer of the mouth.

Occupation and Environment

Many types of industry produce potentially carcinogenic chemicals and by-products, but the severity of the problem is a highly controversial question because of its political and economic implications. In America, estimates of the prevalence of occupation-linked cancers range from 1 per cent to 20 per cent. Some scientists warn that there is a growing epidemic of cancers caused by industry and its effluent. Even the conservative estimate of 4 per cent produced by British epidemiologists Peto and Doll carries the implication that 20 per cent of cancers in manual workers, the most exposed group, are associated with their jobs. The higher estimates calculated by such scientists as Samuel Epstein of Chicago University imply that the majority of cancers among manual workers could be linked with their work.

The most severe problems now seem to be associated with the petro-chemical industry. Areas of generally high cancer prevalence have been found near many large oil refineries including the Avonmouth area in South-West England, and parts of the North-East. In America, a recent survey of counties where the chemical industry is concentrated revealed that men in these areas had excessively high mortality rates from cancers of the bladder, lung and liver. Salem County, New Jersey, leads in bladder cancers; one in four of the employed people in this area work in the chemical in-dustry.

We can be sure that the problem is associated with unrecognized, as well as known, carcinogens. When a hazard takes decades to become obvious, new chemicals and processes are bound to be thought safer than they are in reality. Many types of industrial cancer are now prevented – though perhaps more because of the changes in types of industry and the products we use than because of deliberate action. Examples include the disappearance of cancers of the groin caused by soot – the first recognized work-place carcinogen; also the cancers of the groin and skin caused by mineral oil used to spray cotton-spinning machines in Lancashire; the leukaemias and other cancers induced in radium workers and others who worked with radio-activity before its dangers were recognized. Asbestos is now controlled, as is vinyl chloride, another bladder carcinogen, though how effective such controls are is always a matter of debate.

143

While workers who are frequently exposed to high doses of carcinogens are most at risk, the problem is rarely confined to this population group. Their families may be at risk from contaminated clothing brought home from the factory. The whole neighbourhood may be at risk from fumes and effluent dispersed into the surrounding environment. Disasters like Bhopal and Seveso remind us of the horrors of chemical contamination of whole towns; but we should not ignore the inevitable toll of illness produced by places like the coking plant at Mountain Ash, South Wales, or incinerators dotted all over the country. Even crematoria are probably contributing to their trade through burning plastic-lined coffins, producing dioxins and other poisons.

To reduce the risk of carcinogenesis from environmental and industrial contamination, we have to change our attitudes to the environment. It is becoming increasingly difficult to move away from sources of carcinogens as the countryside is sprayed with a multiplicity of chemicals, while street-level air almost everywhere is polluted with vehicle exhaust. Action to fight pollution at every level is essential to prevent cancers.

Intimate Contact

There is increasing recognition of the links between certain virus infections and cancer.

Examples of viral cancers include cervical cancer, caused by the wart virus (and perhaps the herpes virus), and the various cancers which predominate in AIDS sufferers, including B-cell lymphomas, linked with the Epstein-Barr virus, and Kaposi's sarcoma, linked with cytomegalovirus (see Chapter 10). Some leukaemias are caused by virus infection, while hepatitis B is associated with an increased risk of liver cancer.

One thing that the viruses implicated have in common is their mode of spread; all are transmitted by intimate body contact. The behaviour changes necessitated by the AIDS epidemic will therefore give protection against these types of cancer.

144

Sunlight

Most skin cancers have been convincingly linked with sunlight. However, sunlight is also necessary to all of us, so it does not make sense to regard it as a hazard in the same sense as tobacco.

The risk is significant for fair-skinned people living in tropical or sub-tropical regions. The place of highest prevalence is Queensland, Australia, though the Southern USA also has its skin-cancer belt. In Africa, cancers on the legs in men have been linked with the action of sunlight on tropical ulcers – a problem the women avoid by wearing long skirts.

Moderation is the key as far as exposure to the sun is concerned. If you are of Northern stock, with the characteristic pale skin and blue eyes, your skin is not designed to withstand tropical sun for long periods. It is wise, therefore, to keep the body covered much of the time when outdoors. In Europe, the sun does not climb high enough in the sky to cause problems for more than a tiny minority; there is no significant risk in worshipping the limited sun we get in Britain! Sun-beds and other artificial tanning systems are an unknown quantity as far as skin cancers are concerned; they have not been in use long enough for judgements to be made about risks.

PART 3

ENJOYING CONTINUOUS HEALTH

'The requirements of health can be stated simply. Those who are fortunate enough to be born free of significant congenital disease or disability will remain well if three basic needs are met. They must be adequately fed; they must be protected from a wide range of hazards in the environment; and they must not depart radically from the pattern of personal behaviour under which man evolved — for example by smoking, over-eating, or sedentary living.'

Thomas McKeown

In this final part we shall consider aspects of the wider stage upon which human health is placed. We shall be focussing on the effects of our interaction with our shared global environment as we attempt to fulfil our needs from its resources. It is a rare individual who maintains the belief, against mounting evidence, that we have created in any sense a successful relationship with our planet. The evidence for the unsatisfactory nature of this relationship is the generalized decline in human health, even in the richest countries in the world. There are other factors which could be offered as evidence, indeed there is an ever-growing list: the numbers of endangered species, increasing levels of pollution, the rising threats to personal and social security, the increasing stress of life, and so on. Since they all eventually lead back to adverse effects on human health, that becomes the key to both understanding and solving these interrelated problems.

Before looking at specific areas where we need to reconsider, if not radically rewrite, our script to achieve health, we shall consider the role of medicine in health. This offers a summary in miniature of many aspects of the problems we face. It also provides a springboard from which we can launch into the wider environment and the dynamics of our relationship with it.

Imagine we all live and work in a circus. Because the circus feeds and shelters us, most of us have to do some very dangerous things every day to justify our existence. We are prepared to take risks because we believe we need not worry if we fall; others are manning safety nets which will catch us. We are all part of the show, those who walk tightropes and those who work the safety nets. We share the same beliefs: that doing dangerous things is necessary because a circus is like that, and that it is the only way to live – there is no alternative, no life outside the Big Top.

While the circus life has some shortcomings, which we will acknowledge if pushed, we minimize these with the belief that, although some get injured or killed, a similar fate will not befall us. The trouble is that it is only when we fall that the holes in the net come into focus. It is only when we expect to be caught that we see that the net is already overloaded and failing. Those who operate the nets have warned about this, but we preferred to continue doing dangerous things, to spend our money on new costumes, brighter lights and bigger generators. Since the net operators get good wages, and are dependent upon us continuing to put ourselves at risk, their warnings have come to be given and taken as formalities. Anyway there is no shortage of performers . . .

The assumption in our culture is that the provision of the safety net of medical care equals the creation of health. This assumption takes root and is vigorously promoted for many reasons. As individuals we do not like to confront details of the dangers of life, of disease or injury, let alone the reality of our mortality displayed in the continual cycle of birth and death. We are more than willing to assign power and status to professionals in return for being relieved of these responsibilities. In fact we have gone much further. In what has been called the medicalization of society, every circumstance from a cut finger to emotional disturbance is seen as needing medical intervention.

The medical/social contract might be beyond criticism except for two general effects it has produced. The first is manifested by a cultural illusion from which we all suffer. It is this: whenever we talk about 'health', we are in fact discussing its *opposite* – sickness, disease, or illness. Our overreliance on medicine has had the effect of a distorting mirror on our perception; we think health, and illness is reflected back. So deep and widespread is this illusion that it is only in the last decade that we have begun to develop a descriptive language of health (as opposed to illness, which we endlessly describe and catalogue down to the finest molecular detail).

Health is *not* the same as the simple absence of symptoms of illness. Although this is what is commonly regarded as health, it is only the beginning. Health may be seen as a path to the fulfilment of human potential, both individual and social. It is a route we have barely started to explore and map. The World Health Organization has defined health as 'a state of complete physical, mental and social well-being, and not merely the absence of disease or infirmity', and this is a reasonable starting point. But we are inhibited, at times fatally, from exploration while we are blinded by the cultural illusion we have created. Health and illness are very different things; we have to break the mirror to see them as separate and incompatible concepts. Remember the first rule of bicycle riding; head for where you want to go, not for what you wish to avoid. It is little wonder that in concentrating on illness, our culture fails to create health.

The second effect of our social contract is to give medicine an interest in discouraging us from seeing health as a positive concept. There is no malice in this effect; medical professionals are victims of the cultural illusion as much as the rest of us. Nevertheless, at times the discouragement from medicine is active, as when doctors discount the effects of exercise or emotions on health. Mostly, however, it is passive; medical professionals are quite content to wait until people become avoidably ill before they act. To a degree this is because, as part of the contract, we have given health professionals a social position – 'you are a doctor' – rather than charge them with a social function – e.g. 'eliminate heart disease'.

It is only recently that professional bodies, such as the BMA (British Medical Association), have felt the need to make belated critical pronouncements about such things as smoking and alcohol abuse. Only time will tell whether this is the beginning of a new positive direction. For the present, it appears that medicine is content to preside over avoidable epidemics – of heart disease, cancer deaths, and all the other conditions for which it has no effective answer and about which the causes are known – because they are beyond the remit of medicine's current contract.

While medicine has some spectacular successes, these are against a background where indicators of disease in the population at large are increasing. Even diseases medicine has 'mastered', such as tuberculosis with 20,000 cases per annum, linger beyond its reach, maintaining their threat. Yet where individuals are informed and can act, as with smoking, some disease rates drop. Male lung-cancer rates are falling and the increase in heart disease is slowing down, but neither has anything to do with medical treatment.

To claim that everything medicine does is bad or ineffective would be as unbalanced as to believe that it is an omnipotent good. The point is that in our society the medium of medicine has lost its perspective of health. We are also encouraged to be unrealistic in our expectations; because of this, the actual benefits of much of what medicine does are assumed, rather than scientifically established. As a result we get the worst of both worlds. Effective and valuable procedures are starved of resources, while 'glamorous' specialities attract talent and cash.

The national debate about health (illness) care inevitably centres on the allocation of money. The question is sometimes dramatically posed in terms of 'who shall live?'. Such questions are also part of the illusion. We should be asking 'who is avoidably ill, and therefore wasting the skills and resources of treatment?'. The answer to this question is stark: around 80 per cent of the illness suffered in modern society is avoidable. If only a small proportion of this illness was eliminated, the unavoidably sick could have far better treatment within current resources.

The cultural illusion, the reflection of illness when we think health, needs to be destroyed. Health services should become distinct and separate, both in our minds and in reality, from those services devoted to the sick. But to do this we need to consider not just one illusory reflection nurtured between our culture and our perception, but a self-supporting hall of mirrors, each reflecting, to a greater or lesser degree, illusions about the way we live and fulfil our needs. We especially need to disillusion ourselves about the effects of the process our culture has generated. Reappraising our culture is not easy; it could be as painful as the worst scourge we could imagine. This may be appropriate since health is our motivation. Removing the blinkers of medicine may be the first act at the beginning of a long-overdue journey.

Taking the first step will bring disproportionately large benefits. The greatest danger is to remain passive and accepting in the face of the degeneration of our health. Relying on others to provide answers where there may be none, or expecting others to act on your behalf when there may be no common interest, puts your life in the realm of chance. Acting positively for health, individually, socially, and on behalf of our shared global environment, is the only route out of the potentially terminal cul-de-sac of our culture.

Remaining dazzled by the cultural reflection of medicine, or any other social institution, will inhibit our ability to form the attitudes which will allow us to create health. Life is only a limitless concept within carefully defined conditions; once we accept the limits of those conditions, we will inevitably have to take more responsibility for ourselves. In so doing, we have to address much wider questions than the treatment of symptoms, or strategies for coping with infections. We have to look at a range of human needs, and how we can fulfil them without causing harm to others or our shared environment. The following chapters outline some of the questions we need to consider and answer in this context.

Human Needs

The majority of our health problems are generated by the way we fulfil our needs. Beyond a strictly utilitarian idea of need, much of our fulfilment is directed towards satisfying wants, and many of these are not compatible with health.

Individually we may suspect that some of our pursuits have some harmful effects, but we need to earn a living, get to the shops, keep our clothes clean. We repress the intuitive feeling and go along with what is considered normal in our society. Those cultural mirrors keep convincing us it is acceptable. For many, symbiosis with their culture produces a joyful gung-hoism, where any risk is discounted. Volunteers can always be found to carry out the most dangerous or pointless tasks.

Within the human circus many people will perform without a safety net, simply for the applause and approval. Many will perform without an audience, to satisfy needs of their own. And some will perform even though they know they will fall and be injured or killed. There is a streak of self-destruction which runs through us all; in earlier times a willingness to make such sacrifices contributed to the survival repertoire of our species. Today our culture has distorted this quality into an institutionalized perversity.

Whatever we feel about the desirability, or otherwise, of factors which affect our health, we may feel we have little control over them. Choice is felt to be a limited commodity in mass societies. We may be offered dozens of variations of the same product, each distinguishable from the others only by its advertising and packaging, but we are offered little real choice in things which actually influence our lives and may hasten our deaths. While politicians concentrate on the quantity of votes they need, the quality of choice derived from the political process diminishes.

Health, and the choices which lead to it, requires that we establish a belief in individual sovereignty. Our culture encourages us to believe that individuals are actually paramount. It is a belief that bears little weight when the rights of the individual are tested against other interests in our culture; those who maintain the belief are usually those who find no need to test it. Britain, with anachronistic social structures and atrophied political mechanisms, is particularly bad on individual rights. We remain subjects with duties, rather than citizens with rights. As such we have very low self-esteem; we allow ourselves to become potential victims of a variety of self-generated hazards because we do not believe we have the right to resist or object.

The question of rights frequently appears on political agendas. There is a convention of such rights which covers the populations of all EEC countries, and the USA has a written constitution which is intended to guarantee certain inalienable rights to its citizens. The problem is that all such agendas omit the major areas which are hidden by our cultural mirrors. While they subscribe to freedom of speech, none mentions the quality of the air with which you are expected to speak. Any concept of rights which does not address directly the provision of life's necessities is ultimately meaningless.

The rights which are important today are based upon McKeown's classical requirements of health, quoted on page 145. If we accept the sovereignty of the individual, and by implication a right of the individual to health, we need a legally guaranteed right to the following: to pure, unadulterated food; to uncontaminated water; to unpolluted air; to suitable clothing; to adequate housing; to safe, non-polluting transport; to access to medical care; to information on matters which affect us, and to freedom of association and expression.

How we provide access to these rights will depend upon our political philosophy. In the final analysis it does not really matter: our objective must be an inalienable right to all these necessities for everyone. Without this right we will continue to be faced with the unacceptable contradictions which currently plague us – the homeless beyond state welfare, starvation in the richest nations. deprivation beyond the reach of the international community, and the sick maintaining disease to endanger us all.

The acceptance of the right to the freedom of expression does, of course, allow individuals to reject all or any of the other rights. A right is something which cannot be inflicted. So although you may have a right not to walk the circus tightrope, it is usually undesirable that you also have the right to prevent others from so doing, since that would be an infringement of their rights. As a society, we have to ask ourselves to what degree injurious individual behaviour should be tolerated when we all bear the cost of clearing up its results.

Because we have not developed principles to resolve the problem, the questions which arise are always matters of inconclusive debate. Whether an action is a long-overdue reform or an unwarranted imposition on personal liberty will remain a subjective judgement in the absence of guiding principles. The rights we propose above give a background for developing suitable principles.

Such principles require initial differentiation between public and private. In the public domain, any proposal which has the potential for harmful effects should operate on the *minimum acceptable risk* principle. This would mean that it should be assessed on the worst possible eventuality, and if that constitutes an acceptable minimum risk, the proposal would be accepted. At the moment we do the opposite, we work on the basis of maximum acceptable risk, believing that if we can cope with that we will be all right. An eventuality which is not accepted by experts as likely within the scenario they draw of maximum risk is dismissed as 'impossible'. Hence Chernobyl and Three Mile Island. Many decisions, say, in housing or road improvements, could be delegated as at present, provided the basis of the assessment was public and open to question. Things with a high degree of contention and potential long-range effects, like nuclear power stations, should be open to direct referenda, with equal rights of expression to all protagonists. Weighted voting could be given to those who live closest to such hazards.

The principle of minimum acceptable risk has direct effects. It would mean, for instance, that smoking would be banned in public places, since the minimum risk of second-hand smoking is generally unacceptable to many non-smokers. This does not mean that smoking should be banned, for that would be in conflict with our second principle.

The second principle should be that of *maximum acceptable individual liberty*. This is essential since it is unlikely that the first principle could operate without it. Liberty in this sense is a neutral concept; it means people should be free to do things we consider bad as well as those of which we approve. It would mean that we would have to cease our oppression of victimless crime; the resources we devote to censorship and sexual management could be better used. It makes little sense for us to imprison marijuana smokers while advertising for more tobacco addicts, or to oppress heroin addicts while subsidizing farmers to poison us through our food.

We live in a drug-dependent culture. Indeed the nature of humans may be that life would be untenable without chemicals which modify our perception. There is little logic in the way we discriminate between acceptable and unacceptable drugs. However, since all individuals make a choice in the use of drugs, whether alcohol or heroin, it would be far better to ensure that the clear-up costs of addiction were inherent in the costs of the habit. That would at least end society's open-ended commitment to those who choose illness, while giving the suppliers of selected drugs respectable profits. But does it make sense to seize some drug-dealers' profits, while giving tax-payers money to subsidize others?

Between our two principles — liberty and choice, and minumum risk strategies — there would still be those areas of life where risks are unavoidable. Fishing and building are clear examples of industries in which meeting the needs of others involves unavoidable risk for those who carry out the work. Our culture produces another odd picture in its hall of mirrors. Those who choose to damage their health in their private lives are not required to make any special provisions or undergo medical examination. When such people become ill medical care is lavished upon them. On the other hand, those who undertake risk in occupations which benefit society have to bear the cost of insurance, and perhaps prove their fitness. Should they become injured or get killed, such workers are invariably faced with a long and protracted process to get compensation. Those distorting mirrors are at work on our values once more!

Some countries, notably New Zealand and Sweden, have introduced schemes of automatic compensation for accidental injury. The Swedish scheme is limited to medical misadventure, but in New Zealand it covers any accident, regardless of circumstances. In most countries the injured party has to prove negligence against someone before compensation can be considered. When 'someone' is a multinational corporation or the government, the odds are overwhelmingly against the injured party. It is a situation

153

analogous to that faced by objectors to nuclear power; at the inquiry they have pennies against the millions of the nuclear/electric industry.

Such situations are clearly devoid of natural justice. Establishing the sovereignty of the individual, with rights based upon the sanctity of individual health, would lead to long-overdue reforms in the mechanisms which underwrite our complex society. Freedom of expression, whether in courts of law or planning inquiries, should not depend upon access to resources. One way to overcome this would be to make the proposer, who presumably will benefit from the scheme being proposed, responsible for equalizing the expenditure of the opposition.

Reform is a gradual process, and the success of any measure which allows individuals to make choices affecting their health depends upon the first and most necessary step. We need access to unbiased information. There are many areas of life, such as food labelling and the spread of radioactive waste, where health may be directly affected, but we still have to establish that the right to know is reasonable. There are signs that purchasing power in the supermarket is changing the attitudes of food producers, but little sign that our voting patterns are having any influence on the secretive nature of government.

154

Once facts are available it is felt their interpretation will present a morass of confusion for many people. If the average person is not equipped to cope with the basic needs of life in the late twentieth century it is a damning criticism of our concept of education. The fact that we consider such ignorance natural is a product of the hall of mirrors, aided and abetted by the few who derive advantage from the ignorance of the many. From the top of the social hierarchy stability depends upon things staying much as they are. Those who suffer avoidable early deaths or crippling diseases are casualties in the battle for cultural values; there are no innocent bystanders, the weapons of disease are indiscriminate and we are all at risk.

This said, given the nature of people there's no guarantee that more information and proper education would necessarily lead to a greater consensus over contentious questions. Our social response to all matters, whether AIDS or nuclear waste, is rarely direct. It is more like the graduated response of our immune system: starting with warnings and skirmishes, and building up either to match the problem or fail, as the case may be. Because we produce a random response to problems, we need to adopt the two principles given above; applying them universally to need-fulfilment gives our species the best chance of success and survival.

Let us look at areas of basic human need and spell out the implications of the rights and principles we have proposed as essential for human health.

Food. Pure, unadulterated (organic) food is essential for health. The principle of minimum acceptable risk would prevent the use of biocides, drugs and artificial fertilizers which produce the current unwanted mountains of contaminated and de-natured produce.

On the other hand, our second principle, maximum individual liberty, would enable people to eat whatever they chose – providing two conditions were met. Food associated with specific disease should bear the cost of treating that disease – e.g. white bread should be taxed to cover the cost of diverticulitis and some deaths through bowel cancers. And those advertising foods above the minimum acceptable risk should pay an equal amount of money to enable the risks of their products to be advertised.

Uncontaminated Water. The World Health Organization estimates that 80 per cent of the world's diseases may be attributed to contaminated water. This is *not* just a Third World problem. Industry, agribusiness and our attitudes have ensured that most water is contaminated.

The adoption of minimum acceptable risk in both industry and agriculture today would lead to an improvement, but because of the time lag between dumping or run-off and the residues appearing in aquifers, it would be one or two decades before the benefit was noticed. The problem is that in our hall of mirrors it pays farmers to increase fertilizer use to 500 or 600 per cent to gain a five or ten per cent increase in inedible yield. If you then consider that one ton of nitrogen fertilizer requires the consumption of five tons of fossil fuel, the pollution value of inedible grain mountains is staggering. The sooner we stop adding to the contamination cycle the better. Meanwhile political pressure to clean up our water supply is needed.

If people wish to pollute their water, with alcohol or chemical-based drinks, then the same principles which apply to foods with known hazards should pertain.

Unpolluted Air. We have no choice about breathing and, as we have noted in earlier chapters, air is the most common infectious disease vector. As we have also seen, the things we put into the air add considerably to our disease loading. Since air is so basic to us, we should reject the attitudes which allow the common atmosphere to be used as a gigantic dustbin. Application of our first principle would contribute significantly to a solution,

155

but the problem is so widespread that it requires a concerted public campaign.

Every few days in the small town where we live the air is contaminated by someone burning rubbish in their garden. In the past, the traditional bonfire may have been acceptable; today, when it is likely to contain plastic, it should be a criminal offence. Most plastics, unless burned at very high temperature under carefully controlled conditions, produce very toxic fumes. Even when 'ideally' burned they still produce unacceptable levels of pollution. We need to change our attitude to this invaluable part of our shared global environment.

A major source of air pollution is transport and we deal with this below.

Clothing. It may seem odd to insist on this as a right, but despite the general increase in our standard of living, many old people (and possibly those who refuse the right of housing) are not suitably clothed for the winter. Every year the suffering aged appear on TV without warm hats, quilted coats, gloves and suitable footwear. Why? Clothing is the first line of defence against the cold, and it must be made available to all who need it.

156

Housing. Society's current view of housing is short-term. Political expediency in dealing with the mistakes of the past, combined with an inability to keep up with technical developments, means that we waste money and resources while the number of homeless increases.

Our inability to house the population adequately is best seen as a symptom of other unresolved problems, rather than as a problem in itself, although like all symptoms that is how it tends to make itself felt. Our symptomatic response which produces instant slums and tacky breeding boxes on the one hand and allows a free market on the other, is not effective. The question we need to address is this: do we need to hold the fear of homelessness over people today? And if not, on what terms do we remove that fear? This question may be irresolvable at present; our later discussion will illuminate some of the underlying reasons.

We need to take a longer term view of the housing problem. We all value and love the character and style of older houses, yet we build and renovate in ways which will not last, thus perpetuating the problem for future generations. Much is made of the contribution of architecture and design, but in truth housing is designed with little concept of the basic needs of those who will inhabit it. Thus we have the situation of young families on the fifteenth floor and old people in institutional isolation, a certain recipe for depression and despair. We mix housing and industry, and produce the disease hotspots inherent in such proximity. We ignore human needs beyond the superficial, and thus add to stress and degenerative disease. Until we begin designing housing for human need, the major support role of bad housing in producing disease will remain.

Transport. We all want to be somewhere else some of the time, whether it is to visit friends, get the shopping, or take our annual holiday. The problem is the means limits the end; traffic stifles mobility, and tourists destroy what they go to see. Under the onslaught of mass transport, everywhere becomes like everywhere else, and we go further and faster seeking difference but spreading uniformity.

Perhaps we should ask why we need to go somewhere else, why we cannot create what we seek where we are?

For personal health, and many beneficial effects on our environment, we should try to break the habit of slipping behind the wheel (and towards a coronary) every time we have to go somewhere. Here is a rough scale of distance and means we recommend.

157

A round trip of four miles or less (typical of shopping, going to work, or to the station) – walk! We should all walk this distance briskly each day.

For trips of up to ten miles, why not use a bike (or roller skates)? It is good exercise, you can carry considerable loads, and adopt a form of transportation which is excellent for the environment.

Beyond this you may have to use a car, but always consider public transport options. These are usually bad because of our addiction to cars, although in many areas they are improving. If we accept transport as a right, it should also be free. Free public transport would be highly profitable if the reduction in environmental degradation, pollution and health were included in the account. Simple expenditure/income accounting, where the cost of pollution and illness is discounted, is another trick of the distorting mirrors.

Internal combustion engines compete with us for air. Unfortunately, hydrocarbon exhaust fuels a cocktail of toxins into our shared environment. This need not be the case. Exhausts can and should be cleaned up, it just requires a change in attitude. The protest about the cost of such a revolution is based upon the same distortion as that used to hide other transport costs.

Part of the problem of rationalizing transport needs is that we see *our* car in emotional terms. It is our baby, our persona, our sexual charisma, our armour, our compensation for many inadequacies. We need to be more mature about ourselves and our means of self-expression to resolve these problems; until we are, we must resist the vested interests and insist on cleaning up our personal transport act.

Medical Care. We have free medical care, but we have little say in what we get or how it is applied. The NHS amounts to a series of medieval fiefdoms, dominated by specialist interests, bureaucratic management, political intrigue, rigid hierarchies, and a low priority for the needs of the population at large. At times it appears as if patients are seen as an unwarranted hindrance to the smooth running of the system. Despite this there is much of excellence in the medical repertoire. If we were to change the emphasis of the professionals, from holding social positions to solving social problems, there would be much more.

In this area our needs for information and education are paramount. We should not accept medical intervention without being able to give informed consent, not only of the risks and benefits of intervention, but also of all the other possible approaches to problems which are currently outside the medical repertoire. The information is available, but will only be given if it is demanded as a right.

158

Information. Secrecy protects the interests of those who maintain it. In the age of deterrence, secrecy about military defence is illogical; if you wish to deter potential enemies, the more they know about your deterrent, the more effective it will be. In truth, potential enemies usually know about each other's weaponry; secrecy is to keep the defended population in the dark and it is used to allow governments to have their way without too much embarrassment or scrutiny. And when you want to know about a prescribed drug, the lack of information is not for professional or commercial reasons, but to protect the social relationships of those involved.

Information on whatever concerns us is essential. Once more we have to reverse the picture within our culture. If there is any case for withholding information it should be established openly by those wishing to maintain secrecy. Our assumption should be that everything in the public domain is open to inspection. Government and commercial exploitation as we currently experience them may be impossible under these conditions. Look around: we are four minutes from the edge of the apocalypse, and being slowly destroyed by pollution. The need for openness and change is self-evident.

We need to be in a position to *manage* change, not to be the witless victims of it. But management implies purpose, and the purpose should be the benefit of all, a benefit which would show up in health. This is the only precise and accurate mirror of life provisions and the match of culture to the needs of individuals. With adequate information it is unlikely that we would embark on change which would make this worse.

Free Association. People need to interact with each other, to develop and maintain a complex social life. Our culture tells us we do, but reality suggests otherwise. It is not only the old and impoverished who are lonely and isolated. Many of the emotional problems presented to doctors (and tranquil-lized away) are generated by the unsatisfactory nature of our social life. Because most people are unable to live fulfilling lives, over half the popula-tion regularly surrenders to the comforting illusion of TV soaps. It would be interesting (but totally intolerable) to switch off TV and see what happened. Life for many would be unthinkable, but is spending between 30 and 50 per cent of your waking hours in an electronic fantasy land 'life'?

When designing housing and transport systems, we need to give priority to building community into the lives of people. Although we must think and act as sovereign individuals, and many believe the family is our natural unit, in reality we are tribal animals. We need long-term relationships outside our genetic sphere, we need the variety and spontaneity that free association with our fellows brings. Without it much of our human potential remains unawakened or stifled.

159

Free Expression. Those mirrors tell us we have freedom of expression. The primary reason given for standing on the edge of extinction is to protect this freedom. The illusion is maintained only because so few of us ever try to use our assumed freedom. Every state exercises censorship. And where censorship exists, freedom of expression does not. Qualified freedom is only freedom for those who decide the qualifications.

The effect of our cultural assumptions produces a peculiar paradox: free-dom of expression is frequently used to repress freedom of expression. Thus Mary Whitehouse assumes she should be absolutely free to limit the freedom of what people should view on TV. If we could not turn the TV off, we would all have legitimate grounds for action. Similarly, if we were forced to read or listen to things we did not wish to, we would need a campaign to alter an unacceptable situation.

In a multi-ethnic, multi-valued society, where individual sovereignty is already assumed to the degree that people are expected to decide on major, far-reaching questions, the promotion of censorship says much about the psychology of the promotors. Their final refuge is usually to hide behind children, particularly in matters of sex. While there may be grounds for saying that children will find the reality of sex shocking, this concern can be taken to ludicrous extremes – for instance, when one supporter of censorship was worried about very young children seeing women's breasts! Sex shock is similar to that caused by any sudden change, like jumping into cold water. If children are brought up in an environment of sexual openness and honesty they take it, quite naturally, in their stride. As with all secrecy it is the protectors who are expressing their need for protection, and projecting it on to others.

In the words of the multi-national Helsinki Accord on Human Rights, you should be free to see, hear, read and think whatever you like – you should not be free to prohibit that freedom to others.

These rights, and the principles which guide their application, are necessary because in their absence we make ourselves ill.

Much of the recent vogue for healthy living has focussed on the sort of lifestyle options we detailed in Chapter 2. There is no doubt that incorporating the things we recommend into your life will be beneficial. However we should question the situation that forces us to step outside the norms of our society in so many ways in order to create health. Surely if the effects of our culture were compatible with human need, all the factors necessary for human health would be normal rather than remarkable. The diseases we suffer, and the debilitation that increases our susceptibility to infections and cancers are increasingly products of the mainstream normality of our culture. To achieve a healthy society we must realign the mirrors of perception and reality, and change those elements of our culture which work against our best interests.

To succeed in this we have to be clear about our best interests. Whether the progress generated by our culture is desirable depends on how progress is measured. We derive our scales and units from our culture, and these are usually expressed in terms of monetary wealth, or its equivalent in goods or possessions. The trouble is that such indices do not relate to people; a country can claim to be having an economic boom, while 15 per cent are out of work, many of the children in poverty and need, and thousands of the aged dying of neglect. Nations concentrate wealth and resources within institutions, at the expense of subjects or citizens. We have clearly not developed an economic equation designed to satisfy human need, either in the East or the West, yet we are prepared to die, and kill all other life, for our instinctive devotion to the culture in which fate places us.

If progress, in the widest sense, was tangible rather than illusory, our world would be teeming with centres of excellence. These would be of many diverse sorts, every area of human endeavour would be surging forward as individuals exercised their option to pursue various paths to fulfilment. If our technical and scientific expertise, and our ability to manipulate our environment had any real meaning, we should not be contemplating a future where Belfast, Bhopal and Beirut were the future models of life. The truth is that while we win small victories, decline and degeneration are the general trend. Centres of excellence are a vanishing feature of first-hand life for an increasing proportion of the population; addicted to T V, the majority of people are reduced to second- or third-hand experience of such excellence and that is not what living a life which fulfils individual potential should be about.

Why is this so? Behind the domestic political arguments and the international ideological confrontations, one macro-factor is at work. It is the pressure caused by ever-increasing human numbers.

We may like to believe that the clichés of the population explosion do not apply to us; this may be the most dangerous illusion of all. While any nation, region, or community cannot live within the provision of its own resources, it is suffering over-population. It would be more correct to say that somewhere else, less economically or culturally robust people are suffering to fulfil the insufficiencies of such groups. The primary purpose of economic activity is to feed those who cannot directly feed themselves. Despite surpluses of particular crops, mainly polluted and inedible grains and dairy products, few rich developed nations can support their populations without imports. Each nation imports basic commodities from those lower down the economic ladder; at the bottom, usually exporting basics, often food, in exchange for arms and other high-tech power symbols, are those nations containing the quarter of the world's population which is actually starving.

Our ability to maintain a population which cannot be fed from our own resources depends directly on our ability to exploit others in trade. Until we reverse that situation, so that trade becomes an option rather than a necessity, we will rely on the hypocrisy of charity and the well-intentioned efforts of people like Bob Geldof to salve our consciences.

We are forced by our need to trade to subscribe to secondary values which work against our best interests. Competition in trade, instead of cooperation in need-fulfilment, depends upon 'efficiency', which in most areas of life works directly against 'satisfaction'. Eventually, the drive to increasing efficiency develops its own paradox; it eliminates people, whose ends it was intended to serve. Our value system means that economic efficiency is achieved only by discounting social costs in pollution, waste disposal, hidden subsidies, resource dispersal, unemployment and wealth concentration. Ultimately we all pay the price of our illusory values in degeneration and ill-health.

The core of any real political agenda for the future should be a realistic population policy. To change our attitude towards having children, particularly when this is all many women are expected to do, may be our ultimate health, if not survival, challenge. At a more mundane level, the most common vector of all infectious diseases is other people. The higher the density of our population, and the lower our lowest standard of living, the easier we make it for infections.

Stress diseases are endemic in our society. With all our knowledge, talent and command of resources, are we to condemn ourselves to a state of 'normality' consisting of an ever-increasing struggle to get on, characterized by trampling, crushing and depriving others? Ultimately raising ourselves at the expense of others will enmesh us in their failure. By depending upon the impoverishment of others, we mimic the diseases which also depend upon such conditions to maintain the reservoirs from which they emerge to threaten everyone.

Population, resources and disease are global questions. Many experts working on this problem fifteen years ago, when world population was 3,500 millions (today it is 4,800 millions) considered then that numbers were far above the optimum. Yet despite warnings and inevitable effects, we appear incapable of acting on this most basic of all issues; we stare mesmerized into the distorting mirrors of the values we have created and trust to chance. At the corners of many people's vision, an image from the past is beginning to harden into focus; four horsemen are once more riding into our collective consciousness . . .

The population trap develops a dynamic of its own. When large proportions of people are deprived of essential nutrients and sufficient food their physical and intellectual development is curtailed. Such people are alive, but in no position to fulfil their full potential and life becomes reduced to basics: life on the poverty line, a baby a year and premature death. In all situations human numbers prevent the optimization of human values, and in the absence of those values, other cruder forces take over.

An optimum population is one which can be sustained indefinitely, without the disruption of other species. It is a level which will allow other values to be optimized – initially those we have listed as rights. While demographers are estimating that a population of four times the present number is now in sight, ecologists have calculated that we should be aiming for a global population only one quarter of what we have now. In other words, we are heading for a population of 16,000 millions, whereas we should be reducing to around 1,000 millions.

AIDS is forcing us to change our attitudes to sex. If we could take one small step further and also change our attitudes to reproduction, the tragedy this new epidemic has produced may yet have a positive side. All that is needed is for each woman to limit herself to one child, and for men to accept this limitation. If we could go this far, nature and time would do the rest. In a few generations much of the pressure which generates ill-health in the human population and tragedy in the biosphere could be removed.

The choice we face is to accept an agenda for our future with human health as its primary concern, or to allow our faulty autopilot to take us where it will. The indications of the likely outcome of the latter course are not encouraging. Although we may *feel* we have little option other than to suffer the slings and arrows of outrageous fortune, this is not the case, since it is we who make, load and fire the slings and arrows which presently afflict us.

We are dramatically affecting our environment and our evolution. We have to decide whether to do this with a positive purpose for all humanity, or to allow our actions to provide illusory and short-term benefits for a minority at the long-term expense of the majority. If infectious diseases teach us one lesson it should be that, while we all share a common global environment, the minority on whom benefit is focussed are not immune.

While we subscribe exclusively to a competitive ethic in all things, most people will lose. It may be that part of our drive to pollute and degrade our environment is one facet of our competitive nature; those who can stand more contamination and radioactivity, who can survive on de-natured food in impoverished circumstances, will win this perverse game to which we all appear to subscribe. The problem is that improvement requires change, and in many ways we fear that more than we fear anything else. 'Better the devil (we think) we know ...' We are boxed into a further trap of our own making; we rightly fear disruption and change, yet we obviously cannot continue as we are at present. To break out of what may be a terminal impasse we need a new agenda for the future. The future does not just happen, we create it today.

The purpose of our future agenda and debate is this: If we can face up to the reality of our evolutionary involvement and develop a successful strategy, we will survive. If we cannot, we will fail. In an age when infectious diseases are enjoying a fresh evolutionary upsurge, the question we have to decide is which has the superior strategy and understanding, the humans or the viruses?

Ecology as
if People Mattered

Ecology is the science of the interrelationship of all forms of life, and of life with its environment. Its relevance to health is fundamental; it allows us to understand multi-vectored diseases — for example, the relationship between rats and fleas, the environmental conditions which encourage them, and the diseases which then reach humans via the fleas. Ecology also defines the conditions which are required for the health of any species, but while we know a lot about the needs of rats and fleas, we are not very clear about the conditions necessary for healthy humans.

This may be because the human environment is so complex. We have built a socio-cultural environment on top of the biological and physical foundations of our life. Much of our ill-health is rooted in a fundamental difference between these components of our environment. It is a matter of dynamics: the natural bio-physical environment has a dynamic which is in conflict with the dynamic of the socio-cultural environment we have created. This conflict is the source of human degeneration.

The ecology of our natural environment is characterized by cyclic processes. Everything involved in nature is re-used as part of another cycle. There is no waste; it is a self-sustaining dynamic which will continue indefinitely. But the processes our culture depends upon do not contribute to other life-cycles, they are linear rather than cyclic. Consequently they have the opposite effect to natural processes; environs and resources are irretrievably converted, pollution is created, and non-biological or toxic waste dumped. The covert ethic of our culture creates the conditions which are degrading us and all other life-forms.

If we were to acknowledge the needs of nature, each process we initiate would have a beginning which was the end of other cycles, and an end which was the beginning of another. The idea that the planet, our only self-sustaining spaceship, can be casually torn apart, polluted, and contaminated indefinitely and without harm is the grandest and most dangerous illusion our culture maintains. The longer we continue to subscribe to this belief, the nearer we come to a point of no return, when damage will be irreversible.

In this respect the planet is similar to our body. Our immune system keeps the balance in our favour as long as it can. The various cycles of the biosphere will do the same for the planet, maintaining a balance on which all life depends. In the body of the world we are the organism creating the threat and putting the whole system at risk.

In his book, *Gaia: A New Look at Life on Earth*, Jim Lovelock has detailed the hypothesis that all life on Earth reacts with its environment as a self-sustaining whole. The engines of this balance are the biota which are involved in its fundamentals: the bacteria and other microscopic life-forms which modulate oxygen production and exert influence on the climate. How far this hypothesis can be extended depends more on how acceptable it is to our assumptions than to questions of feasibility.

If we accept it totally the resurgence of infectious disease can be seen in a new light. The balancing act of the microsphere may stimulate it to produce pathogens to which we have only one answer: to resume a more harmonious place in the natural scheme of things, and behave ourselves according to the rules, or be removed from the web of life. Refocussing perception in this way brings back a paradoxical reflection from our culture; infectious diseases may not be the result of divine intervention, but if their role in the overall scheme of things is to maintain the balance of life in its totality, it amounts to the same thing.

Ecology as if people mattered requires that we make human culture compatible with human nature. There is a major problem that must be overcome: the pressure generated by the institutions of our culture. Because they are projections of our collective distorted perception, institutional ends are seldom compatible with human ends. In the short term, institutional ends and human ends may appear identical, but in the long term the divergence is revealed. Institutions outlive their creators and grow beyond human scale and control. Simple things illustrate this tendency. As we write, the Department of Health and Social Security, with thousands of employees concerned with the welfare of millions, is shown to be incapable of giving British pensioners butter and meat from the EEC surpluses; the task is simply beyond the institution.

At whatever level human need is expressed, government and corporate institutions fail to acknowledge the problems. They react with public relations, rather than positive action. For them the aim is business as usual, the devotion to 'progress', that archetypal linear concept. In industrial society the only things which get done are those which favour growth, the concept of 'more', which is in accord with the illusions of the linear accounting system of our culture.

We have spent much time in this book on the harm caused by tobacco. While our accounting may be able to estimate the social cost, it has no way of sending a bill. Nor can those people who starve in parts of Africa where land is devoted to growing tobacco put in a claim. Not only is the real cost disguised by discounting these claims, the harmful effects are actually used to enhance the health of the culture. The rising numbers dying from cancer, heart disease, and other tobacco-related diseases provide extra business for medicine and its supply industries, and for undertakers and coffin fabricators. Perversely, the bad health of a nation contributes to raising GNP, but this element of growth has nothing to do with a rising standard of living.

167

Corporate well-being is similarly dependent upon keeping things linear. If business had to pay the real cost of harmlessly disposing of its waste products, it would be less healthy, but humans and the environment would benefit. This would require a conceptual revolution, away from *quantity* towards *quality*, away from throughput to stock. The attitude should be that things must be made to last, and the more irreplaceable the resources used, the longer they should last. With this attitude plastics would have an indefinite *useful* life, rather than spending indefinite time as waste.

At the moment Britain uses the North Sea as a rubbish tip. The pharmaceutical industry, whose PR tells us their efforts are directed to human well-being, has ships in international waters, burning waste that is too toxic to be disposed of on land. What is burned, what the products of incineration are, and where they will end up is not considered important in the linear process of making and selling medicine. Environmental assault does not appear on the balance sheet.

We can be sure, however, that nature is taking account. It will be attempting to deal with the toxic wastes we produce. They will be recycled, turning up in our food chains, perhaps via many dead of other species; they will turn up on our holiday beaches, or in the bracing sea breezes. For nature does not subscribe to the idea that something can be 'thrown away'; it is all here and now, and we cannot avoid it.

Much of the damage to human health is traceable to the activities of the chemical industry. These multinational corporations have fingers in all the harmful pies, from petro-chemicals through agricultural chemicals to pharmaceuticals. Their activities are harmful because they are linear, rather than cyclic. These businesses take carbon-based molecules, usually from earlier life-forms, and adapt them by compounding them with other substances. They are then released into the environment and given another shot at life, out of time, out of place and out of phase. Some substances so produced, like DDT, leap at the chance; this chemical does everything it can to get into living tissue. Bury it and it resurfaces, drown it and it swims into diatoms, burn it and it floats free; it only rests in living tissue, where it is toxic.

We have a choice. Either we order our affairs so that our processes complement nature, so that our products ultimately become valuable parts of other life-cycles, or we can continue as at present and leave nature to do it for us. If we take the first option, we can live with the rest of the biosphere in some sort of harmony. If we opt for the latter we may be the harmful by-product which nature, in its wisdom, eliminates.

Pollutants in the Home

Discover the household pollutants that could disrupt your immune competence by doing this questionnaire. Arm yourself with a notepad and pen and check your home room by room.

1. Count all the aerosol sprays in your home.
   a) Check your personal items – hair sprays, deodorants, medicines, shaving-cream etc.: how many aerosol cans are there?
   b) Now check fabric-care sprays such as starch, dry-cleaning and proofing products. How many of these?
   c) How many spray polishes and cleaners?
   d) How many spray paints, varnishes, and dyes?
   e) How many cans of air freshener or room deodorizer?
   f) How many cans of fly spray, pet flea spray, household insecticide spray?
   g) Do you use any other sprays in the kitchen – e.g. coatings for cooking vessels? How many of these?

2. Do you use washing powder that contains enzymes (that means almost all types except pure soap, Ecover, or Original Non-biological Persil)?

3. Do you use products which leave your clothes perfumed (including fabric conditioners)?

4. a) Do you regularly wear dry-cleaned clothes?
   b) Does your partner wear dry-cleaned clothes?
   c) Are any of your furnishings dry-cleaned?

5. Do you use long-lasting or block deodorizers (e.g. in the lavatory or kitchen)?

6. Do you use long-lasting insecticides (e.g. Vapona)?

7. Do you use insecticidal pet shampoo, or does your pet wear a flea collar?

8. Do you use strong-smelling glues (such as Evostik) in the house?

9. Is there any new paint in the house (painted within six weeks)?

10. Do you have formaldehyde-urea cavity foam insulation in the walls of your home?

11. Has the timber in your home been treated with preservative within the past year?

12. Do you have plastic-covered furniture?

13. Do you have flexible plastic clothing, shower curtains, tablecloths, etc.?

Now check the places you regularly go outside: the garage, garden shed, and car.

14. Do you have a new car?

15. Do you use cellulose paints?

16. Do you use paint or varnish strippers?

17. Is there an air freshener in your car?

18. Do you use pesticides in the garden?

Finally, back in the house, check your heating and cooking facilities.

19. Do you have gas heaters or a gas cooker?

20. Do you use paraffin or bottled-gas heaters?

Now check your chemical contaminant rating:

Question 1: All aerosol sprays are capable of causing problems. Count 2 for each you find.
Question 2: Add 5 for biological washing powder.
Question 3: Occasional use, add 2; regular use, add 5.
Question 4a: Add 2 for each day during the past fortnight when you wore clothes dry-cleaned within a month.
4b: Add 1 for each day your partner wore recently dry-cleaned clothes in the past fortnight.
4c: Add 2 per item of furniture, carpets, curtains dry cleaned within the past six months.
Question 5: Add 2 per item.
Question 6: Add 5 per item.
Question 7: Add 2 per flea collar, 2 per use of shampoo within the past six weeks.
Question 8: Add 4 for each use within the past six weeks.
Question 9: Add 4 for each room re-painted within the past six weeks plus 4 if you did the painting.
Question 10: Add 10 if yes.
Question 11: Add 20 if yes.
Question 12: Add 10 for furniture less than one year old; 2 per item more than one year old. (Count only flexible coverings.)
Question 13: Add 4 per item less than one year old, 2 per item over one year old.
Question 14: Add 4 for a car less than one year old.
Question 15: Add 6 for each use within past six weeks.
Question 16: Add 6 for each use within past six weeks.
Question 17: Add 2 if yes.
Question 18: Add 2 for each type.
Question 19: Add 20 if you can smell gas anywhere in the house. And whether or not you can smell gas, add 2 for every gas heating or cooking appliance.
Question 20: Add 2 for every bottled-gas or paraffin heater.

171

Now check your rating:

Over 140
Your home is heavily contaminated with chemicals. Check which sources are most significant and start working immediately on eliminating them.

You are over-anxious about dirt, pests and natural smells. Perhaps you take undue notice of the heavy advertising that is designed to make you buy, buy, buy? Remember that a chemical 'fresh' smell is likely to be damaging to your health and use your nose to judge the hazard. Anything you can smell is present in the air you breathe, and it goes straight into your bloodstream from the membranes of your nose and lungs.

A chemically coated surface may be germ-free and it may look good – but that doesn't make it clean, or healthy.

If you've been doing a lot of painting and house renovation, you will have been exposed to a heavy chemical load and you may not be willing to stop the work yet. Protect yourself by keeping the house, car, garage or shed very well ventilated. Leave all the doors and windows open as much as you can; let fresh air waft the poisons away.

172

90 to 140
The chemical contamination level of your home is high and is likely to cause you problems if you are at all susceptible. Probably you have a heavy loading from some sources and little problem with others. Think about why you use so many chemicals: is it convenience, ignorance of their dangers, an over-conscientious attitude to cleaning and polishing?

Now you've been alerted to the major sources of chemical contaminants in your home environment, you will be more aware of them. Throw away as many as you can; stop using others; go back to methods of cleaning that your grandmother might have used.

40 to 90
You are not an excessive user of chemicals but you still have more sources of contamination in your home than you really need. Whether they prove a problem to you depends on your personal sensitivity; you might be reacting very badly to particular sources so that the limited range in your home still represents too much for your detoxifying systems.

Focus on any products that make you sneeze or feel in any way unwell, and get rid of them. Then gradually reduce your use of other potential sources of problems.

Under 40

The level of contamination in your home is well below average, and it may not represent a problem for you unless you are sensitive to particular sources.

If, however, you suffer from any allergies, especially hay fever or asthma, you will need to look critically at every single item that contaminates the air you breathe. The chances are that you can get rid of most of them without much difficulty.

Appendix 2

Exercise

Warning: Do not undertake any of these activities if you are in any doubt about your general level of fitness.

Exercises suitable for extending metabolic capacity include the following:

Running – vary your pace, do not settle into a monotonous jog.

Cycling – get a good bike and use it hard.

Rowing – the real thing has many advantages, but rowing machines are good; avoid the sort with springs.

Swimming – good exercise, but it is difficult to sweat; use swimming for an occasional change of routine.

Roller skating – running on wheels, you will need to spend longer to achieve the same effects.

Beware of plateauing. After an initial phase of effort, you will adapt to your activity; once this happens, the benefits diminish. Try something different, or extend yourself so that you continue to increase your capacity.

Other activities suitable for avoiding plateauing are those which will increase your strength. Try to incorporate some of these into your life once you feel ready:

Canoeing

Digging – grow your own organic vegetables

Football
Gymnastics
Weight-lifting
Hill walking – why not try back-packing some long-distance paths?

Bibliography

Chapter 1

Blackley, C. H., *Hayfever: Its Causes, Treatment and Effective Prevention*, (London: Baillière, 1880).

Deaux, G., *The Black Death*, (London: Hamish Hamilton, 1976).

Doll, R. and Peto, R., *The Causes of Cancer*, (Oxford: Oxford University Press, 1981).

Epstein, S., *The Politics of Cancer*, (San Francisco: Sierra Club Books, 1978).

Hoyle, F. and Wickramasinghe, N. C., *Diseases from Space*, (London: Dent, 1979).

Johnson, C. and Melville, A., *Hay Fever: No Need to Suffer*, (London: Corgi, 1985).

Office of Population Censuses and Surveys, *General Household Survey 1985*, (London: HMSO, 1987).

Stanley, N. F. and Joske, R. A., *Changing Disease Patterns and Human Behaviour*, (New York: Academic Press, 1985).

Wilson, D., *Penicillin in Perspective*, (London: Faber and Faber, 1976).

World Health Organization, *Rift Valley Fever: An Emerging Human and Animal Problem*, (Geneva: WHO, 1982).

Chapter 2

Adam, K. and Oswald, I., 'Sleep Helps Healing', *British Medical Journal*, 24 November, 1984.

Ashton, H. and Stepney, R., *Smoking: Psychology and Pharmacology*, (London: Tavistock, 1982).

Bland, J. (ed.), *Medical Applications of Clinical Nutrition*, (New Canaan: Keats, 1983).

Bryce-Smith, D. and Hodkinson, L. *The Zinc Solution*, (London: Century-Arrow, 1986).

Doll, R. and Peto, R., *The Causes of Cancer*, (Oxford: Oxford University Press, 1981).

Doull, J. *et al.* (eds), *Casarett and Doull's Toxicology: The Basic Science of Poisons*, (London: Macmillan, 1980).

Epstein, S., *The Politics of Cancer*, (San Francisco: Sierra Club Books, 1978).

Erlichman, J. *Gluttons for Punishment*, (London: Penguin, 1986).

Fry, J. 'The Place of Primary Care', in *Trends in General Practice*, (Royal College of General Practitioners, 1979).

Gear, A. *The New Organic Food Guide*, (London: Dent, 1987).

Hanssen, M. *E for Additives*, (Northampton: Thorsons, 1984).

Lynch, J. J. *The Broken Heart: Medical Consequences of Loneliness*, (New York: Basic Books, 1977).

Melville, A. and Johnson, C., *The Long-life Heart*, (London: Century, 1985).

Melville, A. and Johnson, C. *Persistent Fat and How to Lose It*, (London: Century, 1986).

Phillips, M., 'Why Smoking, Not Health, Wins the Day'. *Guardian*, 6 May 1980.

Simonton, O. C., Matthews-Simonton, S., and Creighton, J. L., *Getting Well Again*, (New York: Bantam Books, 1978).

Sterling, P. and Eyer, J., 'Biological Basis of Stress-related Mortality', *Social Science and Medicine*, vol. 13E, (1981), 3–41.

US Department of Health, Education and Welfare, *Smoking and Health: A Report of the Surgeon General*, DHEW Publication no. (PHS) 79–50066, 1979.

Walker, C, and Cannon, G., *The Food Scandal*, (London: Century, 1985).

Warburton, D., 'Nicotine and Smoking', *Reviews on Environmental Health*, vol. 5, (1985) 344–90.

Watts, J., *An Investigation Into the Use and Effects of Pesticides in the UK*, (London: Friends of the Earth, 1985).

Chapter 3

Ader, Robert (ed.), *Psychoneuroimmunology*, (New York: Academic Press, 1981).

Bryce-Smith, D. and Hodkinson, L., *The Zinc Solution*, (London: Century-Arrow, 1986).

Gillman, A. G. *et al.* (eds), *Goodman and Gillman's The Pharmacological Basis of Therapeutics*, 6th Ed., (London: Macmillan, 1980).

Roitt, I. M., Brostoff, J., Male, D. K., *Immunology*, (Edinburgh: Churchill Livingstone, 1985).

Stites, D. P. and Stobo, J. D. (eds), *Basic and Clinical Immunology*, 4th Ed., (New York: Lange Medical Publications, 1982).

Chapter 4

'Risk Factors for Human Immunodeficiency Virus Seropositivity Among Children in Kinshasa, Zaire', *The Lancet*, 20 September 1986.

Ader, Robert (ed.), *Psychoneuroimmunology*, (New York: Academic Press, 1981).

Ball, D., 'Black Lungs and Black Walls', *New Scientist*, 12 February 1987.

Doll, R. and Peto, R., *The Causes of Cancer*, (Oxford: Oxford University Press, 1981).

Epstein, S., *The Politics of Cancer*, (San Francisco: Sierra Club Books, 1978).

Erlichman, J., *Gluttons for Punishment*, (London: Penguin, 1986).

Fraumeri, J. F. (ed.), *Persons at High Risk of Cancer*, (New York: Academic Press, 1975).

Fritsch, A. (ed.), Center for Science in the Public Interest, *The Household Pollutants Guide*, (New York: Anchor Books, 1978).

Gillman, A. G. *et al.* (eds), *Goodman and Gillman's The Pharmacological Basis of Therapeutics*, 6th Ed., (London: Macmillan, 1980).

Glaser, R., *The Body is the Hero*, (London: Collins, 1977).

Grant, E., *The Bitter Pill: How Safe is the 'Perfect Contraceptive'?* (London: Elm Tree Books, 1985).

Hanssen, M., *E for Additives*, (Northampton: Thorsons, 1984).

Millstone, Erik, *Food Additives: Taking the Lid Off What We Really Eat*, (London: Penguin, 1986).

Nicolson, R. S., Association of Public Analysts' Surveys of Pesticide Residues in Food, 1983, *Journal of the Association of Public Analysts*, vol. 22, (1984) 51–7.

Nixon, P. G. F., 'Take Heart', *The BMA Book of Executive Health*, (London: Times Books, 1979).

Parry, W. H., *Communicable Diseases*, 3rd Ed., (London: Hodder and Stoughton, 1979).

Roitt, I. M., Brostoff, J., Male, D. K., *Immunology*, (Edinburgh: Churchill Livingstone, 1985).

Rose, C., *Pesticides: The First Incidents Report*, (London: Friends of the Earth, 1985).

Royal College of General Practitioners, *Morbidity Statistics From General Practice, 1981–2, Third National Study*, Office of Population Censuses and Surveys, (London: HMSO, 1986).

Stites, D. P. and Stobo, J. D. (eds), *Basic and Clinical Immunology*, 4th Ed., (New York: Lange Medical Publications, 1982).

Taylor, B. *et al.*, 'Breast Feeding, Eczema, Asthma, and Hayfever', *Journal of Epidemiology and Community Health*, vol. 37, (1983) 95–9.

Travis, A., 'Deaths From Leukaemia "Twice Expected Figure"', *Guardian*, 17 February 1987.

Vessey, M. P. and Gray, M., *Cancer Risks and Prevention*, (Oxford University Press, 1985).

Watts, J., *An Investigation Into the Use and Effects of Pesticides in the UK*, (London: Friends of the Earth, 1985).

Wood, C., 'Marriage, Separation and the Immune System', *New Scientist*, 24 April 1986.

Wynn, M. and Wynn, A., *Prevention of Handicap and the Health of Women*, (London: Routledge and Kegan Paul, 1979).

Ziff, S., *The Toxic Time Bomb*, (Northampton: Thorsons, 1984).

Chapter 5

McKeown, T., *The Role of Medicine*, (London: The Nuffield Provincial Hospitals Trust, 1976).

Scheff, T. J., 'Decision Rules and Their Consequences', *Behavioral Science*, (1963) 97–107.

Stewart, G. T., 'Toxicity of Pertussis Vaccine: Frequency and Probability of

Reactions', *Journal of Epidemiology and Community Health*, vol. 33, (1979) 150–6.

Taranger, J., 'Mild Clinical Course of Pertussis in Swedish Infants Today', *The Lancet*, 12 June 1982.

Wynn, M. and Wynn, A., *Prevention of Handicap and the Health of Women*, (London: Routledge and Kegan Paul, 1979).

Chapter 6

ASH (Action on Smoking and Health), *Fact Sheet no. 4: Tobacco and Respiratory Diseases*, (London: ASH, 1983).

Office of Population Censuses and Surveys, *Deaths by Cause, 1985*, (London: OPCS, 1986).

Parish, P., *Medicines: A Guide for Everybody*, 5th Ed., (London: Penguin, 1986).

Roitt, I. M., Brostoff, J., Male, D. K., *Immunology*, (Edinburgh: Churchill Livingstone, 1985).

Stanway, A., *Prevention is Better . . .* (London: Century, 1986).

Chapter 7

British Medical Association and Pharmaceutical Society of Great Britain, *British National Formulary*, (The Pharmaceutical Press, 1986).

Erlichman, J., *Gluttons for Punishment*, (London: Penguin, 1986).

Inglis, B., *The Diseases of Civilisation*, (London: Hodder and Stoughton, 1981).

Parry, W. H., *Communicable Diseases*, 3rd Ed., (London: Hodder and Stoughton, 1979).

Paul, A. A., *et al.*, *The Composition of Foods*, (London: HMSO, 1978).

Trowbridge, J. P. and Walker, M., *The Yeast Syndrome*, New York: Bantam Books, 1986).

Chapter 8

Parry, W. H., *Communicable Diseases*, 3rd Ed., (London: Hodder and Stoughton, 1979).

Rowan, R. L. and Gillette, P., *The Gay Health Guide*, (Boston: Little, Brown and Co., 1978).

Chapter 9

Acheson, E. D., 'AIDS: A Challenge for the Public Health', *The Lancet*, 22 March 1986.

Ancelle, R., *et al.*, 'Long Incubation Period for HIV-2 Infection' (letter), *The Lancet*, 31 March 1987.

Carne, C. A., *et al.*, 'Prevalence of Antibodies to Human Immunodeficiency Virus, Gonorrhea Rates and Changed Sexual Behaviour in Homosexual Men in London', *The Lancet*, 21 March 1987.

Eales, L.-J. *et al.*, 'Association of Different Allelic Forms of Group Specific Component with Susceptibility to Clinical Manifestation of Human Immunodeficiency Virus Infection', *The Lancet*, 2 May 1987.

Gallo, R. C., 'The AIDS Virus', *Scientific American*, vol. 256, January 1987, 38–61.

Lyons, S. F., *et al.*, 'Survival of HTV in the Common Bedbug', (letter), *The Lancet*, 5 July 1986.

Morgan, W. M. and Curran, J. W., 'Acquired Immunodeficiency Syndrome: Current and Future Trends', *Public Health Reports*, vol. 101, no. 5 (1986), 459–65.

Osborn, J. E., 'AIDS and the World of the 1990s: Here to Stay', *Aviation, Space and Environmental Medicine*, vol. 57 (1986), 1208–14.

Pinching, A. J., 'Clinical and Immunological Aspects of the Acquired Immune Deficiency Syndrome and Related Disorders', *J. Hosp. Infect.*, vol. 6 (supp.), (1985) 1–8.

Pinching, A. J. and Weiss, R. A., 'AIDS and the Spectrum of HTLV/LAV Infection', *International Review of Experimental Pathology*, vol. 28, (1986) 1–44.

Stewart, G. J. *et al.*, 'Transmission of Human T-cell Lymphotropic Virus Type III (HTLV-III) by Artificial Insemination by Donor', *The Lancet*, 14 September 1985.

Tatchell, P., *AIDS: A Guide to Survival*, (London: Gay Men's Press, 1986).

Voeller, B., 'AIDS Transmission and Saliva' (letter), *The Lancet*, 10 May 1986.

Zuckerman, A. J., 'AIDS and Swimming Pools', *British Medical Journal*, 26 May 1985.

Chapter 10

Blanks, S. and Woddis, C. *The Herpes Manual*, (London: Settle and Bendall, 1983).

Wickett, W. H., *Herpes: Cause and Control*, (London: Futura, 1983).

Chapter 11

Blackley, C. H., *Hayfever: Its Causes, Treatment, and Effective Prevention*, (London: Ballière, 1880).

Hanssen, M., *E for Additives*, (Northampton: Thorsons, 1984).

Johnson, C. and Melville, A., *Hay Fever: No Need to Suffer*, (London: Corgi, 1985).

Mackarness, R., *Chemical Victims*, (London: Pan, 1980).

Mackarness, R., *Not All in the Mind*, (London: Pan, 1976).

Middleton, E. *et al.* (eds), *Allergy: Principles and Practice*, 2nd Ed., (St Louis: Mosby, 1983).

Ministry of Agriculture, Fisheries and Food, *Report of the Working Party on Pesticide Residues* (1982–5), (London: HMSO, 1986).

Royal College of General Practitioners, *Morbidity Statistics from General Practice, 1981–2, Third National Study*, Office of Population Censuses and Surveys, (London: HMSO, 1986).

Royal College of General Practitioners, *Trends in Morbidity in General Practice*, Royal College of General Practitioners, Occasional Paper No. 3, 1976.

Royal College of Physicians and British Nutrition Foundation, 'Food Intolerance and Food Aversion', *Journal of the Royal College of Physicians*, vol. 18, (1984) 83–123.

Steel, M., *Understanding Allergies*, (London: Consumers' Association, 1986).

Taylor, B. *et al.*, 'Breast Feeding, Eczema, Asthma, and Hayfever', *Journal of Epidemiology and Community Health*, vol. 37, (1983) 95–9.

Wadsworth, M., *Inter-generational Differences in Child Health*, Office of Population Censuses and Surveys, Occasional Paper 34, (1985) 51–8.

Chapter 12

Bunyard, P. and Searle, C., 'The Effects of Low Dose Radiation', *The Ecologist*, vol. 16, no. 4/5, 1986.

Doll, R. and Peto, R., *The Causes of Cancer*, (Oxford: Oxford University Press, 1981).

Epstein, S., *The Politics of Cancer*, (San Francisco: Sierra Club Books, 1978).

Forbes, A., *The Bristol Diet*, (London: Century, 1984).

Fraumeri, J. F. (ed.), *Persons at High Risk of Cancer*, (New York: Academic Press, 1975).

Meirik, O. *et al.*, 'Joint National Case-control Study in Sweden and Norway', *The Lancet*, 20 September 1986.

Millstone, Erik, *Food Additives: Taking the Lid Off What We Really Eat*, (London: Penguin 1986).

Office of Population, Censuses and Surveys, *Deaths by Cause, 1985*, (London: OPCS, 1986).

Stites, D. P. and Stobo, J. D. (eds), *Basic and Clinical Immunology*, 4th Ed., (New York: Lange Medical Publications, 1982).

US Department of Health, Education and Welfare, *Smoking and Health: A Report of the Surgeon General*, DHEW Publication no. (PHS) 79–50066, 1979.

Vessey, M. P. and Gray, M., *Cancer Risks and Prevention*, (Oxford: Oxford University Press, 1985).

Chapter 13

Antonovsky, A., *Health, Stress and Coping*, (New York: Academic Press, 1982).

Dubos, R., *Man Adapting*, (New Haven: Yale University Press, 1965).

Dubos, R., *Man, Medicine and Environment*, (London: Pall Mall Press, 1968).

Meadows, D. H., Meadows, D. L., Randers, J., Behrens, W. W., *The Limits to Growth*, (London: Pan, 1974).

Index

189

FOR THE BEST IN PAPERBACKS, LOOK FOR THE

In every corner of the world, on every subject under the sun, Penguin represents quality and variety – the very best in publishing today.

For complete information about books available from Penguin – including Pelicans, Puffins, Peregrines and Penguin Classics – and how to order them, write to us at the appropriate address below. Please note that for copyright reasons the selection of books varies from country to country.

In the United Kingdom: For a complete list of books available from Penguin in the U.K., please write to *Dept E.P., Penguin Books Ltd, Harmondsworth, Middlesex, UB7 0DA*

In the United States: For a complete list of books available from Penguin in the U.S., please write to *Dept BA, Penguin, 299 Murray Hill Parkway, East Rutherford, New Jersey 07073*

In Canada: For a complete list of books available from Penguin in Canada, please write to *Penguin Books Canada Ltd, 2801 John Street, Markham, Ontario L3R 1B4*

In Australia: For a complete list of books available from Penguin in Australia, please write to the *Marketing Department, Penguin Books Australia Ltd, P.O. Box 257, Ringwood, Victoria 3134*

In New Zealand: For a complete list of books available from Penguin in New Zealand, please write to the *Marketing Department, Penguin Books (NZ) Ltd, Private Bag, Takapuna, Auckland 9*

In India: For a complete list of books available from Penguin, please write to *Penguin Overseas Ltd, 706 Eros Apartments, 56 Nehru Place, New Delhi, 110019*

In Holland: For a complete list of books available from Penguin in Holland, please write to *Penguin Books Nederland B.V., Postbus 195, NL–1380AD Weesp, Netherlands*

In Germany: For a complete list of books available from Penguin, please write to *Penguin Books Ltd, Friedrichstrasse 10 – 12, D–6000 Frankfurt Main 1, Federal Republic of Germany*

In Spain: For a complete list of books available from Penguin in Spain, please write to *Longman Penguin España, Calle San Nicolas 15, E–28013 Madrid, Spain*

THE PENGUIN COOKERY LIBRARY – A SELECTION

The Best of Eliza Acton Selected and Edited by Elizabeth Ray
With an Introduction by Elizabeth David

First published in 1845, Eliza Acton's *Modern Cookery for Private Families*, of which this is a selection, is a true classic which everyone interested in cookery will treasure.

Easy to Entertain Patricia Lousada

Easy to Entertain hands you the magic key to entertaining without days of panic or last minute butterflies. The magic lies in cooking each course ahead, so that you can enjoy yourself along with your guests.

French Provincial Cooking Elizabeth David

'It is difficult to think of any home that can do without Elizabeth David's *French Provincial Cooking* . . . One could cook for a lifetime on the book alone' – *Observer*

The National Trust Book of Traditional Puddings Sara Paston-Williams

'My favourite cookbook of the year. Engagingly written . . . this manages to be both scholarly and practical, elegant without pretension' – *Sunday Times*

The New Book of Middle Eastern Food Claudia Roden

'This is one of those rare cookery books that is a work of cultural anthropology and Mrs Roden's standards of scholarship are so high as to ensure that it has permanent value' – Paul Levy in the *Observer*

FOR THE BEST IN PAPERBACKS, LOOK FOR THE 🐧

COOKERY IN PENGUINS

Jane Grigson's Vegetable Book   Jane Grigson

The ideal guide to the cooking of everything from artichoke to yams, written with her usual charm and depth of knowledge by 'the most engaging food writer to emerge during the last few years' – *The Times*

More Easy Cooking for One or Two   Louise Davies

This charming book, full of ideas and easy recipes, offers even the novice cook good wholesome food with the minimum of effort.

The Cuisine of the Rose   Mireille Johnston

Classic French cooking from Burgundy and Lyonnais, including the most succulent dishes of meat and fish bathed in pungent sauces of wine and herbs.

Good Food from Your Freezer   Helge Rubinstein and Sheila Bush

Using a freezer saves endless time and trouble and cuts your food bills dramatically; this book will enable you to cook just as well – perhaps even better – with a freezer as without.

An Invitation to Indian Cooking   Madhur Jaffrey

A witty, practical and delightful handbook of Indian cookery by the much loved presenter of the successful television series.

Budget Gourmet   Geraldene Holt

Plan carefully, shop wisely and cook well to produce first-rate food at minimal expense. It's as easy as pie!

COOKERY IN PENGUINS

Mediterranean Food   Elizabeth David

Based on a collection of recipes made when the author lived in France, Italy, the Greek Islands and Egypt, this was the first book by Britain's greatest cookery writer.

The Vegetarian Epicure   Anna Thomas

Mouthwatering recipes for soups, breads, vegetable dishes, salads and desserts that any meat-eater or vegetarian will find hard to resist.

A Book of Latin American Cooking   Elisabeth Lambert Ortiz

Anyone who thinks Latin American food offers nothing but *tacos* and *tortillas* will enjoy the subtle marriages of texture and flavour celebrated in this marvellous guide to one of the world's most colourful *cuisines*.

Quick Cook   Beryl Downing

For victims of the twentieth century, this book provides some astonishing gourmet meals – all cooked in under thirty minutes.

Josceline Dimbleby's Book of Puddings, Desserts and Savouries

'Full of the most delicious and novel ideas for every type of pudding' – *Lady*

Chinese Food   Kenneth Lo

A popular step-by-step guide to the whole range of delights offered by Chinese cookery and the fascinating philosophy behind it.

FOR THE BEST IN PAPERBACKS, LOOK FOR THE

COOKERY IN PENGUINS

The Beginner's Cookery Book   Betty Falk

Revised and updated, this book is for aspiring cooks of all ages who want to make appetizing and interesting meals without too much fuss. With an emphasis on healthy eating, this is the ideal starting point for would-be cooks.

The Pleasure of Vegetables   Elisabeth Ayrton

'Every dish in this beautifully written book seems possible to make and gorgeous to eat' – *Good Housekeeping*

French Provincial Cooking   Elizabeth David

'One could cook for a lifetime on this book alone' – *Observer*

Jane Grigson's Fruit Book

Fruit is colourful, refreshing and life-enhancing; this book shows how it can also be absolutely delicious in meringues or compotes, soups or pies.

A Taste of American Food   Clare Walker

Far from being just a junk food culture, American cuisine is the most diverse in the world. Swedish, Jewish, Creole and countless other kinds of food have been adapted to the new environment; this book gives some of the most delicious recipes.

Leaves from Our Tuscan Kitchen   Janet Ross and Michael Waterfield

A revised and updated version of a great cookery classic, this splendid book contains some of the most unusual and tasty vegetable recipes in the world.

GARDENING IN PENGUINS

The Penguin Book of Basic Gardening   Alan Gemmell

From the perfect lawn to the flourishing vegetable patch: what to grow, when to grow and how to grow it. Given the garden, a beginner can begin on the day he buys this book with its all-the-year-round Gardener's Calendar.

The Pip Book   Keith Mossman

All you need is a pip and patience . . . 'The perfect present for the young enthusiast, *The Pip Book* should ensure that even the most reluctant avocado puts down roots and sends up shoots' – *The Times*

The Town Gardener's Companion   Felicity Bryan

The definitive book for gardeners restricted by the dimensions of their gardens but unrestrained by their enthusiasm. 'A fertile source of ideas for turning a cat-ridden concrete backyard into a jungle of soothing green' – *Sunday Times*

Water Gardening   Philip Swindells

A comprehensive guide to the pleasures and uses of expanses of water, however great or small in the garden. Includes advice on aquatic and marginal plants and the management of ornamental fish.

Beat Garden Pests and Diseases   Stefan Buczacki

An invaluable book, covering all types of plants, from seedlings to root vegetables . . . there is even a section on the special problems of greenhouses.

The Englishman's Garden   Alvide Lees-Milne and Rosemary Verey

An entrancing guided tour through thirty-two of the most beautiful individual gardens in England. Each garden is lovingly described by its owner. Lavishly illustrated.

A History of British Gardening   Miles Hadfield

The great classic of gardening history. 'One of the most interesting, stimulating and comprehensive books to have come my way. It should be on every gardener's bookshelf . . . a remarkable book' – Cyril Connolly in the *Sunday Times*.

Roses for English Gardens   Gertrude Jekyll and Edward Mawley

Illustrated with beautiful photographs, this book demonstrates the nearly limitless possibilities for planting the best-loved flower of all – between walls, on pergolas, along wood posts, on verandas, and on trees.

Labour-Saving Gardening   Tom Wright

At last, a guide to make sure that you get maximum pleasure from your garden – with the least effort and just a little forethought and planning. Every aspect of gardening is investigated – all to save your most precious commodities: your energy and your time.

Gardens of a Golden Afternoon   Jane Brown

'A Lutyens house with a Jekyll garden' was an Edwardian catch-phrase denoting excellence, something fabulous in both scale and detail. Together they created over 100 gardens, and in this magnificent book Jane Brown tells the story of their unusual and abundantly creative partnership.

Window Boxes and Pots   Martyn Rix

Patio, balcony or windowsill – all can be transformed into an eye-catching delight with this wonderfully informative guide. Whether you settle for lobelia cascading from a hanging basket or geraniums of white, soft pink and cosy scarlet, you can be sure that Martyn Rix will tell you all you need to know.

Audrey Eyton's F-Plus   Audrey Eyton

'Your short-cut to the most sensational diet of the century' – *Daily Express*

Caring Well for an Older Person   Muir Gray and Heather McKenzie

Wide-ranging and practical, with a list of useful addresses and contacts, this book will prove invaluable for anyone professionally concerned with the elderly or with an elderly relative to care for.

Baby and Child   Penelope Leach

A beautifully illustrated and comprehensive handbook on the first five years of life. 'It stands head and shoulders above anything else available at the moment' – Mary Kenny in the *Spectator*

Woman's Experience of Sex   Sheila Kitzinger

Fully illustrated with photographs and line drawings, this book explores the riches of women's sexuality at every stage of life. 'A book which any mother could confidently pass on to her daughter – and her partner too' – *Sunday Times*

Food Additives   Erik Millstone

Eat, drink and be worried? Erik Millstone's hard-hitting book contains powerful evidence about the massive risks being taken with the health of consumers. It takes the lid off the food we eat and takes the lid off the food industry.

Pregnancy and Diet   Rachel Holme

It *is* possible to eat well and healthily when pregnant while avoiding excessive calories; this book, with suggested foods, a sample diet-plan of menus and advice on nutrition, shows how.

PENGUIN HEALTH

Medicines: A Guide for Everybody   Peter Parish

This sixth edition of a comprehensive survey of all the medicines available over the counter or on prescription offers clear guidance for the ordinary reader as well as invaluable information for those involved in health care.

Pregnancy and Childbirth   Sheila Kitzinger

A complete and up-to-date guide to physical and emotional preparation for pregnancy – a must for all prospective parents.

The Penguin Encyclopaedia of Nutrition   John Yudkin

This book cuts through all the myths about food and diets to present the real facts clearly and simply. 'Everyone should buy one' – *Nutrition News and Notes*

The Parents' A to Z   Penelope Leach

For anyone with a child of 6 months, 6 years or 16 years, this guide to all the little problems involved in their health, growth and happiness will prove reassuring and helpful.

Jane Fonda's Workout Book

Help yourself to better looks, superb fitness and a whole new approach to health and beauty with this world-famous and fully illustrated programme of diet and exercise advice.

Alternative Medicine   Andrew Stanway

Dr Stanway provides an objective and practical guide to thirty-two alternative forms of therapy – from Acupuncture and the Alexander Technique to Macrobiotics and Yoga.

A Complete Guide to Therapy   Joel Kovel

The options open to anyone seeking psychiatric help are both numerous and confusing. Dr Kovel cuts through the many myths and misunderstandings surrounding today's therapy and explores the pros and cons of various types of therapies.

Pregnancy   Dr Jonathan Scher and Carol Dix

Containing the most up-to-date information on pregnancy – the effects of stress, sexual intercourse, drugs, diet, late maternity and genetic disorders – this book is an invaluable and reassuring guide for prospective parents.

Yoga   Ernest Wood

'It has been asked whether in yoga there is something for everybody. The answer is "yes" ' – Ernest Wood.

Depression   Ross Mitchell

Depression is one of the most common contemporary problems. But what exactly do we mean by the term? In this invaluable book Ross Mitchell looks at depression as a mood, as an experience, as an attitude to life and as an illness.

Vogue Natural Health and Beauty   Bronwen Meredith

Health foods, yoga, spas, recipes, natural remedies and beauty preparations are all included in this superb, fully illustrated guide and companion to the bestselling *Vogue Body and Beauty Book*.

Care of the Dying   Richard Lamerton

It is never true that 'nothing more can be done' for the dying. This book shows us how to face death without pain, with humanity, with dignity and in peace.